Out in the Open

The Complete Male Pelvis

Out in the Open

The Complete Male Pelvis

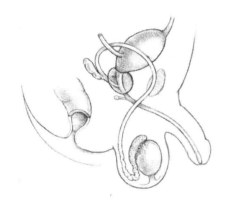

R. Louis Schultz, Ph.D.

Photographs by Sean Kahlil

Illustrations by Lauren Keswick

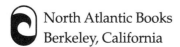

North Atlantic Books
Berkeley, California

Out in the Open: The Complete Male Pelvis

Published by
North Atlantic Books
P.O. Box 12327
Berkeley, California 94712

Cover photo by Sean Kahlil
Cover and book design by Paula Morrison

Printed in the United States of America

Out in the Open: The Complete Male Pelvis is sponsored by the Society for the Study of Native Arts and Sciences, a nonprofit educational corporation whose goals are to develop an educational and crosscultural perspective linking various scientific, social, and artistic fields; to nurture a holistic view of arts, sciences, humanities, and healing; and to publish and distribute literature on the relationship of mind, body, and nature.

Library of Congress Cataloging-in-Publication Data

Schultz, R. Louis (Richard Louis) 1927–
        Out in the open : the complete male pelvis / R. Louis Schultz :
    photographs by Sean Kahlil ; illustrations by Lauren Keswick.
        p.   cm.
    Includes bibliographical references and index.
    ISBN 1-55643-321-2 (alk. paper)
    1. Generative organs, Male—Anatomy.   2. Pelvis—Anatomy.   3. Body image in men.   4. Masculinity.   5. Men—Attitudes.   I. Title.
QM416.S38   1999
611'63—dc21   99-16525
                                                                     CIP

1 2 3 4 5 6 7 8 9 / 03 02 01 00 99

Dedication

To the headless models who patiently allowed photographs of their very private areas.

Acknowledgments

The author is deeply indebted to Sean Hellier, without whose computer expertise and patience this book would probably never have been put together. I am also grateful to him for the extensive web search he did on the subject of circumcision.

Considering the subject of circumcision, it was very difficult to determine who does what where. It occurred to me that probably nowhere in the world is there a greater variety of cultures and nationalities than among New York City taxi drivers. So I asked many of them about that custom in their country. They were all extremely informative, and many were interested in my findings. One Chinese driver was so enthused about having been circumcised after he came to the U.S. that I was afraid he was going to show me his penis. Fortunately, heavy traffic prevented that.

I am grateful to Rosemary Feitis, D.O., my co-author of *The Endless Web*, for her comments on the organization of the material in this book.

I wish to thank those who have read through the manuscript and made helpful suggestions and criticisms—Tom Divan, Tom Groenfeldt, Michael Orton, and Marcelo Coutinho.

Rolfing® is a registered trademark of the The Rolf Institute of Structural Integration.

Table of Contents

List of Illustrations

Preface

TOUCHING BODIES IS A VERY INTIMATE EXPERIENCE—especially when it is intimacy without sexual context. Much of the insight in this book comes from my twenty-five-plus years as a bodyworker. Not only does the client's body relax and open up, but the other aspects of one's life history—emotions, negative and positive body memories, inhibitions, family and cultural relationships—all can emerge. This may be especially frightening to a man. To these insights, I have added seventy-plus years of living as a man in many situations and environments. This book is not about Rolfing, it's about men....

Although this book is not intended specifically for bodyworkers, there are some rather detailed anatomical descriptions, mainly to identify the physical relationship between the anus and the genitals in men and some of the unconscious emotional consequences of rigidity. This is something I have not found discussed elsewhere. There is also a section for bodyworkers on how to safely work in the pelvic area.

Over the years, I began to realize how we men accept the stereotype of being insensitive to our feelings. It is dogma that women talk about their feelings with each other and men don't; the sexual manuals have summed up the same conclusion. What do I mean by men's feelings? I looked up the word "feeling" in the dictionary. It reads as follows: *capacity to feel; sense of touch; physical sensation; emotional reaction; particular sensitivity; intuition or notion; general sentiment; sympathy; compassion; emotional sensibility or intensity; sensitive; heartfelt.* When I refer to men's feelings, I mean any and all of these.

I came into Rolfing from a strictly scientific background—Ph.D. in physiology, teaching anatomy in medical school, research in embryology and reproductive physiology. In that world, any published studies based on testimonials were considered unscientific. I no longer believe that numbers and statistics are the only valid data.

In 1972, I was on sabbatical in California—the days of the Humanistic Psychology Movement—and I wanted to experience that. The real reason for my going to a Rolfer was life-long back problems. During every one of the first ten sessions, I laughed so hard that my Rolfer had a difficult time not breaking up himself. After the sessions were completed, I felt cheated. The expected emotional breakthroughs—tears, anger, fear—that were supposed to happen during the process had not happened to me. Then I realized that the joy and laughter were my emotional releases.

The memory (which came later) was that when I was young my father worked nights and slept during the day. I had a very loud laugh—it was called a "cackle." My mother reproached me about my laughter waking up my father. From then on for approximately thirty-five years, I literally did not laugh. It was frequently commented, "You smile a lot, but you never laugh." The laughter that was released was a belly-laugh—I had released the long-held tension in my abdomen and other parts of my body to allow that happy response.

Another effect of the work was that I became more athletic than I had ever been in my life. My sports activities had always been curtailed by my bad back. All of this was enough for me to quit the restrictive academic life and become a maverick bodyworker.

Rolfing gave me the confidence to trust my intuition about myself and other men and to acquire a language to express it. I do not consider myself a therapist. I'm a good listener and have the ability to relate a comment from one person to that from another and to still another, until I have some kind of complete understanding. Through all of this, my sense of humor has allowed me to see the drama we live with.

My life experience has been varied. I have lived in a number of cultural environments—the Mid-west, the Pacific Northwest, northern and southern California, the Rocky Mountain region, Belgium, and the Big Apple. Body-watching has been my hobby for all of my life, especially the male body, since I think we all do comparisons. Although my work has been on both men and women, this book is about my revelations of working with, listening to, and watching men—the things men don't talk about.

My teaching and bodywork knowledge of men's bodies comes from all parts of the U. S., Germany, France, England, Italy, Belgium, Switzerland, Brazil, and three territories in Australia. The cultural attitudes of men toward their bodies was quite different in each country, yet I noticed similarities in physical protection. My amusement in these countries was to study the typical movement of local men's bodies and attempt to relate it to their culture.

It has been my privilege to have a number of male protégés who have contributed to my awareness of the attitudes of younger men of various ages and cultures. Their love and respect has been a most positive influence in my life's journey.

Following is a compilation of observing, researching, discussing, intuition, hearing, seeing, smelling, touching, arguing, agreeing, disagreeing, thinking, wondering, teaching, exploring inwardly, and other exploring physically, emotionally, and mentally that has been done over more than twenty-five years of bodywork plus more than seventy years of living as a Scorpio. Much of my own life experience is in this book.

Introduction

FIRST TRAINED AS A ROLFER (see Appendix I) over twenty-five years ago. I began the work filled with good intentions of bringing balance and harmony to the bodies and the lives of anyone who was willing to submit to my hands and limited knowledge. After six months, a teacher of mine, Judith Aston, reviewed the Polaroid® photos that I had taken of my clients after each session. She commented that each of my clients looked different before they started the process. Midway through, they started to look the same—compressed in the groin area. This was especially true of my male clients. I looked at myself in the mirror and saw that I was also "short" (compressed) in that part of my body.

I realized that I was afraid to touch that part of a man's body. One fear involved the possibility of causing damage. Another fear was the possibility of the client misunderstanding my intention. Shortly after Judith's comments, I had the opportunity to do a dissection on a male body with several other Rolfers. I paid special attention to the structure of the pelvis to find out what was safe to work on and what was not. I will admit that no one else was allowed to touch that pelvis: I wanted to be absolutely sure that nothing was cut away before I had a chance to look at it.

Structural protection in the male cannot be understood without considering possible reasons for such protection, both physical and mental. The first and most obvious consideration is the external positioning and sensitivity of the genitals. The fear of being injured in the testicles would cause a pulling in, both consciously and unconsciously. The unconscious is the most interesting since it would begin very early in the male infant.

Less obvious are effects of the moral and cultural values with which the man is raised. In the northern cultures especially, men are ashamed of their feelings. Men don't cry. Pleasure and joy are not part of the vocabulary. Sensual is considered feminine. Erotic must be immoral. The biggest problem with these attitudes is that the messages are generally non-verbal. Such messages are hard to be conscious of, much less to rebel against. This necessitates being more aware of what a man "doesn't say," or listening for the little side comments that he will make from time to time about his feelings and/or his background. Such awareness can start while doing the body work and then spill over into the bodyworker's personal life.

This awareness opened a pathway of observing and understanding general patterns of males' protection of the pelvic region. This area is generally not discussed by men, who say very little about their genitals except, in some cases, to brag about their sexual prowess and, in fewer cases, about their penis size. The anus is not discussed at all. A direct question to a man about what he feels in his pelvis is usually met with embarrassed silence or a change of subject.

Doing bodywork on many men has offered me an opportunity to observe similarities and differences in the male pelvic structure. Working in the pelvic area makes clear the areas of sensitivity (don't touch). There is a general pattern of protection both structurally and functionally in the groin region, whether the genitals hang low between the legs or are positioned more "up front." Working around the coccyx (tailbone) usually results in a tight clamping of the entire buttocks, and some men (if they can verbalize it) complain that they feel as though their anus is being penetrated. The latter demonstrates how insensitive a man can be in the anal area and brings up the fears of anal penetration.

My concern was that my information was coming from an older generation (mainly, my own). I have noted that the protective structural restrictions are similar in the pelvis of men of various ages and cultures. My question was whether the reasons were the same. In an attempt to get input from men of different ages and cultures, I gave an outline of this text to a variety of my male clients, friends and casual contacts and asked for reactions. The usual initial response was very little comment (frequently, "very interesting"). On later visits, more response occurred. It

seemed as though they needed time and permission to be O.K. with thinking about their own pelvic area. An occasional comment was, "Men don't
talk about this."

One of the best sources has been women, especially mothers of boys.
Their openness demonstrated that they knew what was going on during
their son's early development even though the boys had no idea that their
mothers were aware. Some fathers preferred to live in oblivion about their
son's maturation.

Many of my observations are intuitive and guesswork based on min-
imum explicit output from others. Dr. Rolf used to say that intelligent
guesses are valid.

1

General Observations

THE EASIEST WAY TO BEGIN TO UNDERSTAND the structural tightness and protection of the male pelvis is by observing the way the pelvis moves when the man moves. This will vary to some extent from culture to culture. Although the focus here is on the pelvis, obviously the entire body is involved with any movement. The ideal situation is when any one part of the body moves, the entire body responds.

Before considering structural and movement patterns that are unique to the male structure, it is necessary to look at those patterns that exist in both men and women. Movement will affect body structure and body structure will affect movement.

There are four general body structural patterns. There are two extreme patterns. One is a forward curve in the lumbar region (lordosis) with the pelvis tilted forward, creating a rounded buttocks. The extreme opposite is a flat lower back with the pelvis tilted backward, usually associated with a flat butt. Two less common patterns can occur—a flat rear with a curved lower back or a rounded buttocks with a flat lower back (Fig. 1-1). Genetics probably accounts for the basic patterns. I have a suspicion that people may modify their body carriage in an unconscious attempt to blend into their environment—much as accents can change in a new location.

An additional consideration in body structure is whether the weight of the upper body is carried in front of the hip joint or behind it. The

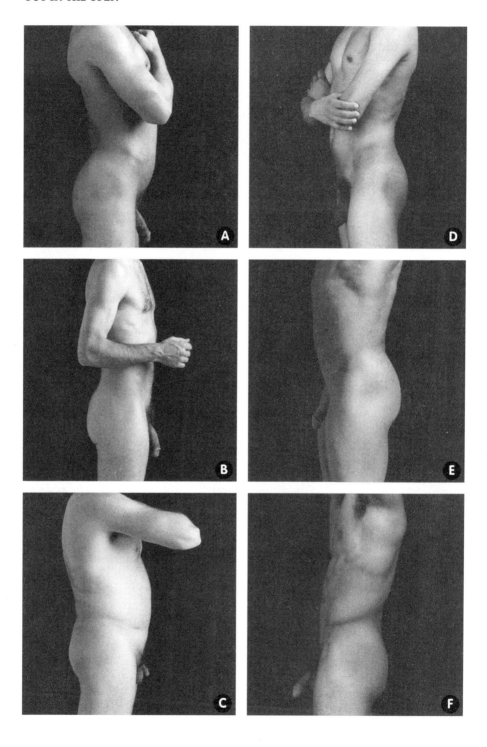

weight in front of the hip joint will give the impression of the legs being dragged from behind. With the weight behind the joint, the legs look as though they are being pushed forward by the body weight. The curved back is generally related to the forward shift of the body weight, the flat back to the backward shift. Again, the reverse can occur (Fig. 1-1). The body patterns become a problem only when they are exaggerated and cause discomfort. One of the focuses of Rolfing is to help the person's weight become positioned over (on top of) the femurs.

The position of the femur (thigh bone) in the hip socket will influence the position of the legs and the movement of the pelvis. When the femurs are rotated medially (inward) in the joint, the knees are turned inward and the legs bow outward—postural bowlegs. In lateral (outward) rotation of the femurs, the knee caps are facing outward and the legs are pushed together—postural knock-knees. With bowlegs, the tissue of the pelvis is spread wider, giving the appearance of a broader rear end. The movement of the hips is a jerky bouncing from side to side. With knock-knees, the cheeks of the buttocks are pushed together and the movement is an alternating bouncing up and down of the cheeks. These movements are more obvious in men. Pants are more revealing than skirts.

There are modifications of pelvic movement unique to the male body. These relate to the narrower pelvis and the presence of external genitalia. The interaction of cultural, emotional, and physical factors will bring about each man's method of protecting the intimate areas in the pelvis. Over the years of bodywork, I have noted general patterns that seem to occur in the majority of men.

Generalities are always difficult because for every generality, there are dozens of variations. Men with the flat buttocks, back, and neck will often have their body weight behind the center line of their legs. It can be a tucking under of the pelvis, a pushing forward of the genitals, and a sort of throwing forward of the legs—the John Wayne walk. Such men

---

◀ FIGURE 1-1

A side view of six models demonstrating variations in the lumbar curve
(A) is an example of extreme anterior tilt of the pelvis; (C) shows a posterior tilt of the pelvis with the corresponding straight back.

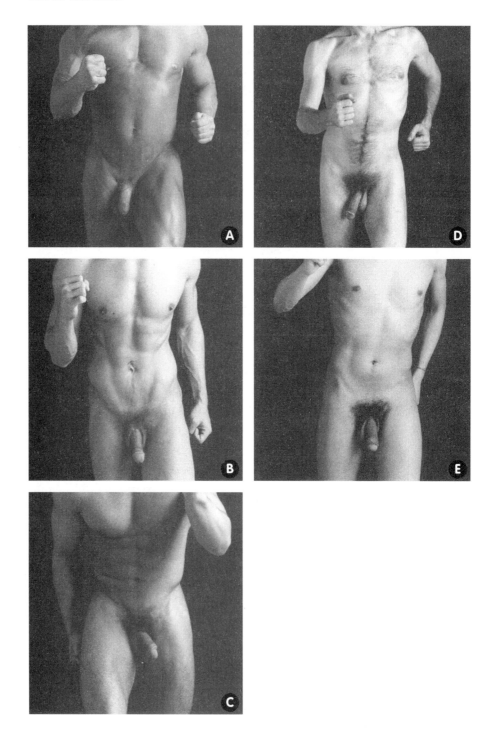

can give the appearance of falling backward.

With the rounded, protruding buttocks, the body weight tends to be placed in front of the femur. Men with this posture may look as though they will fall forward. The appearance is that of pulling the legs forward from behind. The movement is in the hip joints while the back remains "pulled up" (Fig. 1-1).

In some men, the pelvis does not move when they walk. This relates to a tightly held back and abdomen. The trunk of the body resembles a solid block, with arms and legs either being used stiffly like a robot or swinging from the block. Over years of such rigidity, problems inevitably develop in the lower back and the groin area.

A variation is cheeks which are so closely bound together that they rub against each other in walking. This often is seen in men whose body weight is in front of their legs, giving an appearance of falling forward. This can be accompanied by the rubbing together of the upper thighs. It gives the appearance of someone who has the urgency to go to the toilet and cannot. The sphincter muscles (urinary and/or anal) do not feel strong enough, so the muscles of the upper thigh (adductors) are being used in an effort to supplement the sphincters. It's almost as though the person is walking with crossed legs. This man looks as though he is constantly guarding against having an accident in front or in back, even when the urge or emergency is not there.

There is the image of the man whose pelvis and thighs are used as a single unit. The walk is a swinging from front to back with the movement coming from the lower back. A variation of this is the swinging of the pelvis from side to side (swishing), again with the movement coming from the lower back and with little action at the hip joint. This latter movement seems to be the one most feared (Figs. 1-2, 1-3, 1-4).

I remember a TV ad for something or other which showed a muscular young man doing aerobics with a group of young women. He went

---

◄ FIGURE 1-2
Simulated walking, front views
(A) and (C) move the pelvis like a block with no pelvic rotation; in (B) and (D) the pelvic girdles are elevated over the back leg.

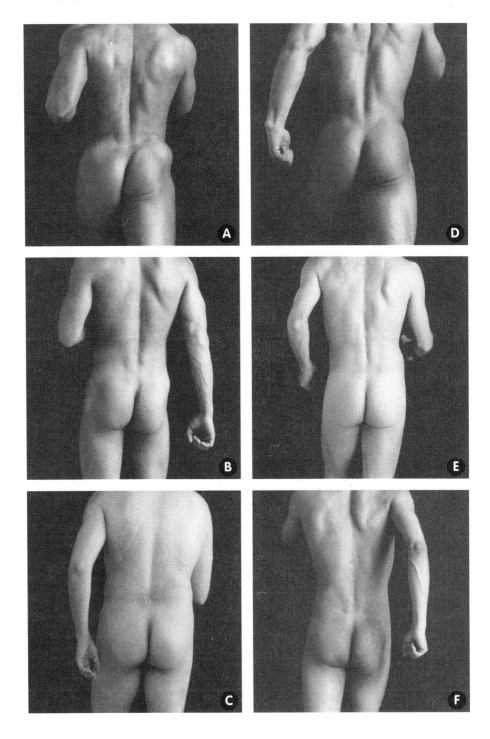

with the group in the exercise until the movement of the pelvis from side to side was called for. At this point he threw up his hands and walked away. It was summarized dramatically that he didn't do that movement because "He was a man." This demonstrated the mentality and attitudes of manliness on the part of the advertisers and what they felt the public would like and relate to.

Viewed from the front, it is common for men to look as though they are walking around their genitals. This means that when they walk, their genitals remain quiet—not moving. It is as though the body were composed of three columns. The outer two columns move while the center one, with the genitals at the bottom, does not. This gives a sort of strut to their gait. A much smoother walk can occur when the body is used as two columns with the movement going through the genitals. Perhaps the fear here is that of being too sexy, too feminine, or too suggestive.

Many men I have worked with tell me that they simply cannot move their pelvis (i. e., they hold it stiff) in a public situation, especially at work. The fear stems from the concern of being misunderstood. Or, the fear may be that of feeling good about one's self and one's body in that situation, a feeling of vulnerability. One man worked for a large corporation. He did not feel comfortable allowing his pelvis to move in front of his co-workers so he practiced his walking in empty halls. Another young man worked on a construction crew. He said any pelvic movement at work would result in cat-calls, whistles, and sexual references. He practiced his pelvic movement away from the job.

The defense of the pelvis becomes more apparent with touching. Almost any touch on or around the buttocks will cause the response of tightening of the buttock muscles and a pulling in of the anal sphincter. This is especially true when the touch is around the tailbone or the "sitz" bones (tuberosities). This can be related to the fear of being "unclean."

◄ FIGURE 1-3

Simulated walking, back views

(A) and (D) demonstrate extreme tightness in the lumbar muscles and the rubbing together of the gluteal muscles; some tightness of the cheeks is apparent in all models with the least in (E); (C) has basically no movement in the pelvis.

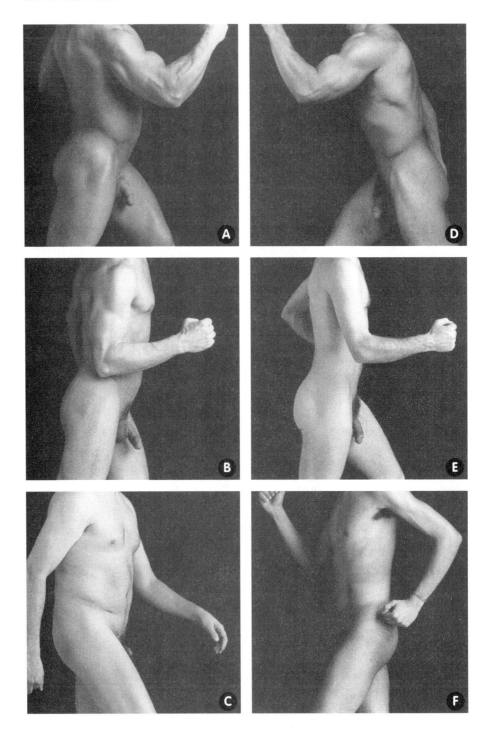

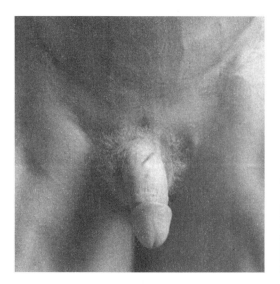 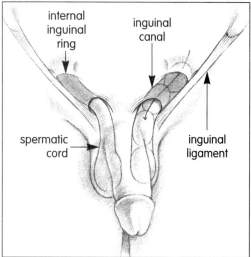

FIGURE 1-5
Pathway of descent of testicles prior to birth
Internal inguinal ring is exit point of testicle from abdominal cavity.

How many of us have been criticized or ridiculed by our mothers for yellow or brown spots on our underwear?

In front the sensitivity to touch is below the waistline. The breath does not go down to that area, indicating a lack of feeling—emotion, physical sensations, or both (see Appendix II). The groin area (inguinal) is especially touchy, often painful (Fig. 1-5). Anger can be displayed when that area is touched. The fear can be that of getting aroused in a non-sexual situation (or of not getting aroused in a sexual situation). It seems that it is acceptable to have the capacity to feel the penis at the appropriate time, not in the area surrounding it at any time. The image I often have is that of the penis sticking through a tight girdle. This can relate to men's lack

◄ FIGURE 1-4
Simulated walking, side views
(C) and (F) walk with the body leaning back; (B) and (D) are leaning forward; (A) appears to be leaning forward with an anterior tilt of the pelvis, yet the shoulders are held back, shortening the lower spine; (E) is walking the most in line.

of awareness of the emotionally motivated feelings in their bodies, about their sensual feelings in general, and especially about sensitivity in that area.

Just before birth, the testicles leave the safety of the body cavity in the mid-groin or the inguinal region (internal inguinal ring). The testes then migrate down under a layer of very thin tissue in the lower abdomen and descend into the scrotum, where they are suspended by a very thin cord of tissue containing blood vessels, nerves, and the duct to carry the sperm at the appropriate time (Fig. 1-5). The area of exit of the testes in the groin is where so many men are extremely "touchy" (Don't touch me there!). Could it be that this is the area of real castration fears rather than the scrotum? Thus protection of the genitals and that area in general may start in men before birth.

This hypersensitivity would be further complicated in the case of boys with undescended testicles who require surgery after birth. Such surgery results in pain and scar tissue formation and will cause greater desensitization of the area.

2

After Birth

SINCE THE EXTERNAL GENITALIA of the male are indeed external, they are readily available to insult. The delicacy and sensitivity of the genitals are discovered very quickly. In general, subjecting any area to pain will cause a tightening, an internal withdrawal of feeling from that area. This will result in a numbness and desensitization of that area. The testicles especially may be painfully stimulated early on.

Many years ago I was staying with a young couple who had recently had a male child. As often happens with new parents, the discussion turned to changing diapers. The father spoke of how careful he was to clean around the boy's testicles after a bowel movement so as not to hurt him. The mother said something to the effect, "I don't worry about that— I just wipe him off." My thought was, "Of course she's not careful—she doesn't have balls." On later reflection, working with many male clients in the groin region, it occurred to me that most of us were cleaned by our mothers. This could result in an association of hurt testicles and bowel movements and the consequent protection of that area throughout life. This protection (as in other parts of the body which hurt) results in a tightening of the genital/anal region, blocking of feelings, and a resultant "pulling in" of the area. Men will not be aware of the lack of feeling since it starts almost immediately post-birth.

Most mothers (and some fathers) of boys have been extremely defensive when I mentioned this story. They have assured me with indignation that they never hurt their son's testicles. One male client in his forties said that he wished that his wife would be more sensitive to his balls when she played with them. It hurt. He was afraid to mention this to her because he didn't want her to stop the foreplay.

Another factor in early life is circumcision. There has been much emotional discussion and biased research on this subject (see next section). There seems to be no question that there is some pain involved. Many studies have been done on how to diminish the pain. Advocates of painless childbirth believe that circumcision counteracts the environment of comfort that they feel is important after birth. In uncircumcised boys the foreskin adheres very tightly to the head (glans) of the penis, and it should not be drawn back until it is normally loosened—from six months to three years of age. Doing so will tear the tissue and create pain. Either source of pain can cause withdrawal of feeling from the penis and subsequent numbness.

There is the irritation of diapers. They can rub on the sensitive head of the penis, especially if the boy has been circumcised. Since the male pelvis is narrow, bulky diapers may cause the legs to be more splayed out in a manner that might lead to bowlegs. When the diapers are not changed often enough the result can be diaper rash, which will produce unpleasant feelings in the genitals and subsequent withdrawal.

Perhaps more damaging to the psyche are the unspoken or indirect messages. These are the feelings or attitudes of the parents. Often, especially in the older generation, there is the unspoken attitude of the anogenital region being "dirty." This attitude can apply to the body in general.

I do not mean to give mothers a bad rap. Yet, discussions about pelvic problems and attitudes with my male clients and friends most often go back to the mother. The father can also be included in contributing to these problems since he maintains his own rigidities. It can be that the parents are nervous about touching the genital area, especially in a first-born male child. Natural erections that occur may cause discomfort and upset. The natural tendency for the child to touch his genitals will often result in discipline like slapping of the boy's hands and saying, "No, no—that's not nice!"

The concern of sexual abuse by the parents, relatives, or family friends has become more prevalent. It stands to reason that this concern will result in more hesitation about touching the child more intimately. Unfortunately, we may be reverting to less touching in general.

Something I have heard from new mothers of boys is the upset at the "fountain" from the penis when the diaper is removed and air hits the penis. One man related that his family's favorite story is that he peed in his father's face when he was a baby. The penis, of course, is covered with haste, accompanied by some negative comments and attitudes. These verbal and nonverbal responses will certainly imprint on the young child and begin subconsciously to create negative feelings about his genitals. In general, these negative attitudes about the pee-pee will be reinforced by the rest of the family, the community, and the culture.

Still more disapproval centers on the anus. Is there anything more satisfying than a good bowel movement at any age if we relax and allow the feeling? When this happens with babies, the response seems to be almost a sigh of contentment. The response from the adult is anything but positive. If someone other than the mother is holding the baby at that time, there will be a hurried "You take him, you take him!" It becomes clear to the child that he has done something wrong. This pleasure must be bad and subconsciously he must cut off feelings. This will be emphasized if the clean-up is rough and angry.

There are the traumas of toilet training, especially if it is forced at too early an age. A few years before she died, a man's mother proudly told him that he was totally toilet-trained at eight months of age. If she had ever told him that before, he had not registered it. He then remembered his cousin telling him how she had disapproved of his mother disciplining him with a hair brush. He suddenly had a belated understanding of the source of pelvic problems, both physical and sexual, which he had experienced in his life.

Excretion accidents will manifest feelings of shame. What feels natural to the child can cause disgust from others and eventually self-disgust. This is especially true if the child is older."You are a big boy. This happens only in babies!" Of course, the adult has not responded to the timing of the child's needs. In the adult, when a man has "shit" in his pants because of a sudden attack of diarrhea or "peed" in his shorts when a place for relief was not available, the self-criticism and embarrassment can be almost overwhelming.

Self-control becomes the issue—control of bodily functions and control of feelings. This is a matter of degree. To live in society, we all require a degree of control. Too much control, however, and we can become automatons. Control is always being right. Control is not letting your feelings influence your life. Control is not letting the joy of life be a goal. Control is not expressing your feelings. Control is being neutral or neuter. Control is not being sensual. Control is lessening the enjoyment of sex. Control is not being aware of or responsive to the feelings of others since you are not aware of your own feelings. Control is always being on an even emotional plane.

The best way to achieve such control is not to feel, to become numb. This can apply to the entire body and is especially true in the anogenital region. Protection begins by pulling in the offending penis and anus. The breath to the area also becomes restricted.

Since the exhale is the relaxing part of the breath, holding residual air in the body may serve as a buffer against pleasurable or unpleasant feelings. Experiencing a more complete exhale can produce feelings of anxiety and vulnerability. This habit pattern of the incomplete exhale can apply even when urinating or having a bowel movement. Pushing happens with the inhale and holding (naturally one must inhale in order to have something to exhale). The exhale will allow the sphincters to relax and the process will be more efficient and pleasant.

When we are sitting on a toilet seat or squatting in the wilderness, real control becomes relaxing and letting go. How many times have we been in a public restroom where the air is filled with sounds of groaning, straining, and horrendous flatulence coming from the toilet stalls? The reaction is to hold the breath and push rather than breathing and allowing the inner sphincter to relax so that the bowel movement can take place easily. Many people into yoga will stand on the seat and crouch to open the anal sphincter more.

Unfortunately, the concept of control in our society is tightening, holding on. In the case of the bowels, it is appropriate to have control in order not to have an "accident." Holding over too long a time can lead to constipation.

A male flight attendant reported that there is a significantly higher incidence of bladder and urinary tract infections as well as hemorrhoids among his male peers. There can be the factors of rapid change in altitudes, different time zones, and interference of normal sleep patterns. He believed that one problem was the need to refrain from natural eliminations while serving the passengers and again having to wait until the passengers use the toilets after the meals. Such "holding on" on a daily basis could be detrimental to the normal function of the urinary tract and colon.

3

Circumcision

ALTHOUGH THIS TOPIC deviates from the original focus of this book, the general ignorance about circumcision seems to warrant a more detailed description.

I initially considered the concept of circumcision as one of the normal life experiences in the male infant. Yet, on further thought, I realized that the majority of men in the world are not circumcised. The questions arose: who, where, when, and why? Estimates are that about 85% of the men in the world are not circumcised. The country with the highest percentage of men who have had this procedure is the United States. It is the most common surgery performed in this country.

Circumcision is one of the oldest surgical procedures known. It has been practiced for more than 6000 years. One suggestion is that it was present 15,000 years ago in primitive cultures. In the Stone Age, the procedure was performed with flint knives. It is thought that the bleeding which resulted in men simulated the monthly bleeding in women and was part of a ritual.

There is evidence that circumcision was practiced in ancient Egypt, especially among the caste of priests. A drawing on the wall of an Egyptian tomb dated 2400 BC demonstrates the procedure. The ancient Egyptian mummies were circumcised. The practice seems to have arisen independently in various primitive tribes, e. g. some tribes in Africa, many natives in early America, and the Australian Aborigines.

Circumcision is a religious ritual for Jews and Muslims. It comes from Abraham's covenant with God (Genesis 17:9-14) in which the procedure was described. In Judaism, circumcision is a symbolic token, a physical distinguishing mark of Jewishness. It is performed on the eighth day after birth as indicated in the Bible, the Mosaic practice. In biblical times in Egypt, many Jews were not circumcised in order to imitate the Egyptians. Only the Egyptian high priests were relieved of their foreskin. Later, in order for the Jews to enter Palestine, their entry was contingent on their being circumcised. If necessary, circumcision was performed at the border.

The traditional pattern for both Jews and Muslims is to circumcise at a similar time, six to eight days after birth. It has been pointed out that Mohammed never told his followers to be circumcised.

It is generally unknown that circumcision was promoted in the United States in the late nineteenth century as a cure for masturbation. Masturbation was considered to be a cause of many illnesses: madness, idiocy, epilepsy, spinal paralysis and convulsions, a form of insanity, priapism (constant erection), insomnia, blindness, consumption, heart disease, memory loss, and adult suicidal tendencies. It was thought that removal of the foreskin would diminish the pruriency of sexual appetite and result in its cessation. There were tortuous methods of preventing masturbation such as tying the hands, immobilizing the child's body, and other ways to prevent the male child from reaching his penis. In that Victorian time, there was much hysteria about the evils of masturbation.

At about the same time (1870–1890), there were claims from the medical profession that circumcision was a cure for paralysis, serious orthopedic disease, epilepsy, hernia, and lunacy. These were thought to be a result of the nervous consequences of genital irritation by an adherent or constricted foreskin (prepuce). This was a time of surgical experimentation on the genitalia of both sexes to relieve reflex neuroses. (Note: this was also a period of "normal ovariectomy" in women to relieve symptoms ranging from hysteria and neurasthenia to backache.)

Once the circumcision procedure had been established, in the early twentieth century it became a sanitary measure. The concept of personal cleanliness had expanded in the late nineteenth century. Cleanliness became an essential criterion of social respectability. Dirt was seen as a moral and social hazard. Thus circumcision replaced soap and water as a daily routine. New claims were made for the value of removing the foreskin in males. It was said to be a cure for fecal incontinence and constipation. It was considered a safeguard against malignancies such as cancer and syphilis and a prophylactic for impotence.

In the twentieth century, circumcision became a standard practice—a sanitary measure and prophylactic against venereal disease. It became a mark of class distinction as the foreskin came to signify ignorance, neglect, and poverty. Since many of the doctors were Jewish, they tended to encourage the procedure. In time the white, middle-class gentiles accepted the idea and the cost, leaving the recent immigrants, the African-Americans, and the poor with foreskins as a mark of lower class and inferiority. The penis began to be considered "dirty." During World War I (and World War II) circumcision was considered necessary for "hygienic reasons." Some soldiers who refused were disciplined and/or dishonorably discharged. Medical textbooks began showing the circumcised penis.

These concepts spread to the English-speaking countries—England, Canada, Australia, and New Zealand. In 1945, however, the British dropped circumcision from the list of medically insured services and the number of circumcised infants quickly dropped. By 1949, there was a virtual cessation of medically-motivated circumcision in Canada, Australia, and New Zealand.

In the U.S., although routine hysterectomies, tonsillectomies, and gall bladder removals decreased, circumcision increased. It reached its peak in the 1960s and '70s when 85–90% of the male children were circumcised. The benefits of this routine procedure began to be questioned in the 1960s. Could circumcision be a beautification comparable to rhinoplasty? In early 1970s, the American Academy of Pediatrics concluded that there were no medical grounds for routine infant circumcision when comparing the "potential" medical benefits with "inherent" risks and disadvantages. This statement was for the most part ignored by the general medical profession.

Today in many U.S. hospitals, removal of the foreskin on the third or fourth day after birth is routine. The practice appears to be local and regional. In California the number of circumcisions is decreasing. When asked, many parents say they choose the procedure for social reasons—so the son will be like the father and his peers and not subject to ridicule.

There seems to be no question that foreskin removal is accompanied by pain. This has been measured by increased heart rate, increased respiratory rate, and intensity of crying. There is a plethora of literature on studies to reduce the pain of the procedure. General anesthetic is not considered by most to be appropriate since it could result in the death of the child. A dorsal penile nerve block (local anesthetic) is said to be the most effective despite adverse local and systemic reactions. Other methods that have been tried (classical music, intrauterine sounds, sucrose-coated pacifier) have been shown to have no effect on pain reduction.

The literature on the pros and cons of circumcision is filled with emotional debate. Many conclusions have been drawn from incomplete or biased data. The controversy over the value of the foreskin (prepuce) involves medical aspects, religion, esthetics, sexuality, cultural sensitivity, social engineering, psychology, ethics, constitutional rights of the newborn, and cosmology.

The advocates of circumcision present it as a precautionary deterrent to various conditions and diseases. The rationalizations in the Jewish faith are sanitation, an aid to procreation, and a deterrent to sex crimes and intermarriage; the real purpose remains obscure. In the medical rationale, it is accepted (but not proven) that there is a somewhat higher incidence of urinary tract disease in non-circumcised boys the first year. There are some indications that it may be a little higher in circumcised boys after that time. In both situations, the incidence of the disease is relatively rare.

Conditions considered to be prevented by circumcision are: pathological constriction of the foreskin over the glans (head) of the penis [phimosis]; inflammation of the tip of the glans and the foreskin [posthitis]; painful constriction of the glans (head) of the penis by the retraction of tight foreskin behind the head [paraphimosis]; susceptibility to venereal disease; and cancer of the penis in older men. Again, these conditions are rare.

Those in opposition to the procedure make the analogy that circumcision to prevent these conditions is like pulling teeth to prevent cavities. The constriction of the prepuce can be alleviated by making a small slit in the tissue to relieve pressure. Most conditions are considered to be preventable by better education in hygiene. The major complication to the surgery is possible hemorrhage and infection, which if excessive could lead to loss of the tip or entire penis, or to death. Although extremely rare, such disasters have been reported. A condition that has been reported from circumcision is a narrowing of the urinary opening (meatal stenosis), which is a result of ulcerations at the opening of the head of the penis caused by removal of the foreskin.

The foreskin appears in the fetus at two months of pregnancy as a thickened ring of epithelium growing forward over the glans of the penis. By four months, this foreskin has grown over the entire glans, forming a continuous layer adhering to the epithelial covering of the head (Fig. 3-1). The formation of the space between the layers of the foreskin and the head is rarely complete at birth or in the first six months after birth. The foreskin may be non retractable up to three years of age. When this is the case, the suggestion is not to force the foreskin back over the glans until it is structurally ready to do so. It is thought that the foreskin protects the glans from urine and feces. The inner surface of the prepuce is a mucous membrane richly supplied with blood vessels, sensory nerves, and stretch receptors.

In the original description of the procedure as practiced by the Jews, only the outer foreskin, the tip, was removed, preserving the inner lining *(bris milah)*. The practice today by the medical profession is generally more extreme. It starts with breaking the "adhesions" and then applying either a clamp or other device to crush and then excise the tissue of the prepuce. In most cases, the foreskin is removed down to the base of the glans. The baby is restrained and often the face is covered.

Those practitioners who advocate birth without violence strongly oppose circumcision. They consider the practice to be torture, emotional and physical abuse, and sexual abuse. They believe it causes a change in the brain's stress response system. It may cause bonding impairment in the first years of life especially from the pain in the raw penis rubbing against the mother's body while breast feeding.

The following is a distribution of attitudes about circumcision in different countries and parts of the world. These have been accumulated by

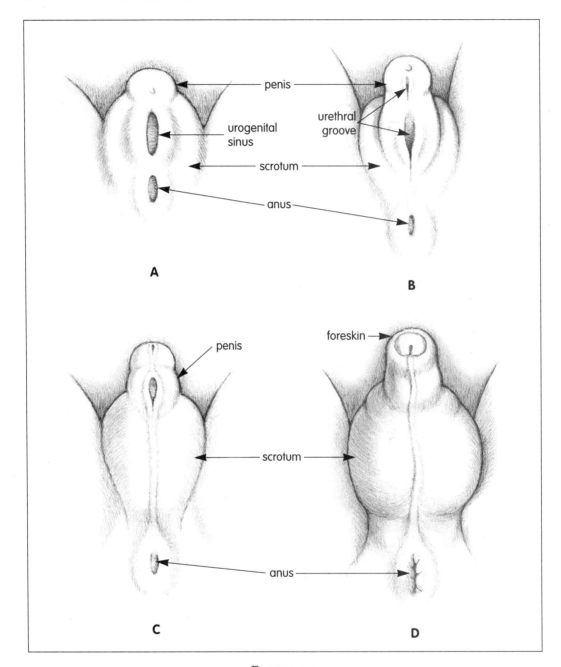

FIGURE 3-1

Stages in the development of male genitalia

Approximate stages of pregnancy: (A) 7th week; (B) 10th week; (C) 12th week; (D) near term

literature search and personal interviews. As indicated previously, circumcision was a common practice in the English-speaking countries until recent years. The United States now is considered to have one of the highest rates. Circumcision is not generally seen in continental Europe, Scandinavia, Japan, or South America. In Spain, I am told, it will happen only if the doctor recommends it, which also seems to be the case in Mexico. In northern Africa, Turkey, and the Near East where the population is mostly Arab (Muslim), it is the general practice. The Muslims are circumcised in India, while the Buddhists and Sikhs are not. In China, circumcision is not generally known except in the province just north of Tibet, where the inhabitants are Muslim.

My information from Argentina is that the church is officially against circumcision and can make it difficult to have the procedure done. In Brazil, there seems to be a class difference, especially in Rio de Janeiro where they try to be more American than the Americans. In central Africa, there is a variation from tribe to tribe. Some tribes have circumcision at puberty as a "rite of manhood." Among some Arab peoples, circumcision is done immediately before marriage. In native Samoa, the boys are circumcised at any age from three to twenty. The followers of Taoism and Buddhism in the Far East rejoice in the intact body.

There is obviously little agreement on the advantages or disadvantages of circumcision. I have talked to a number of men who were circumcised as adults. They are very positive about the results from both a sanitary and cosmetic point of view. On the other hand, there are cases of prepuce reconstruction in circumcised men who felt they had been deprived of a body part without their consent.

The subject is controversial even among adult individuals. Many women and gay men are biased to the point of precluding sexual relations with one or the other (circumcised or uncircumcised men). In the end, the old adage remains true: beauty is in the eye of the beholder.

4

The Juvenile Years

T HE YEARS BETWEEN BABYHOOD AND PUBERTY are the time when boys
become little men. This is especially true for the oldest boy in the
family or an only son. The expectations are high. One way to imitate being a man is to repress feelings. Sometimes such boys are dressed
as little men and subjected to the ridicule of their peers.

There is the confusion of wanting to be like father and also wanting
to blend in with other boys. These efforts are seldom verbalized. It is more
a matter of nonverbal imitation with little positive feedback. You are
expected to do what is appropriate without being told what that is. Negative feedback is freely given.

At this stage, control becomes a greater issue. There is the fear of "accidents" which might occur when the necessity is greater than the control
of the bladder muscles or the anus. Too often young boys become so
involved in their play that they ignore the need for a toilet until it is too
late. This will result in embarrassment, ridicule, shame, and discipline.

Often there is the response of pressing together the inner thigh muscles to reinforce the bladder muscles or the anus. Some adults walk with
the inner thighs permanently clenched so that these muscles actually rub
together. Ways of walking in the adult can be initiated in childhood. I can
remember after my inner thighs were Rolfed, I could literally hear the
sound of corduroy. I had worn corduroy knickers when I was very young
and hated the sound. So I positioned my legs to walk in such a way that

the rubbing of the material would not happen. This adjustment of my thighs became fixed.

Perhaps the greatest trauma for a young male is bed-wetting. I have heard many horror stories about the treatment of this, such as the penis being tied by a string at night, the hands being wrapped at night, or the arms being strapped to the sides of the body. There is the Michael Landon movie drama featuring the mother who hung out the wet sheets with yellow streaks from a front window for the world to see, and how the young boy ran home to take down the sheet before his friends could see it. Sometimes I have observed that men who have a bed-wetting story will have an abnormally small penis. This could be a permanent drawing in of the offending member.

At this stage of physical and emotional development, perhaps the greatest influence comes from peers. Children, like adults, want to blend — to be a part of the group. There is the tendency to imitate body language as well as verbal language and dress. Males from those families where nudity is accepted will often have a problem fitting into their social environment among their peers. They may find that lack of modesty around other boys will produce ridicule or negative comments. One man told me that he went to a summer YMCA camp when he was young. When he walked around the tent naked, one boy commented: "It's not nice to walk around that way." He felt ashamed and after that kept himself covered at all times. Boys may become increasingly uptight, particularly about the anogenital region. This region, if mentioned at all, will be the subject of jokes and distaste.

Many of us will remember the embarrassment and discomfort of enemas. Habitual tightening of the anal sphincters has already been established, probably in the process of toilet training. Therefore, the pushing of the enema tube by an uptight parent into a tight anus will be anything but pleasant and will create further tenseness. This protection could already have been established by the use of rectal thermometers in the baby.

The passing of gas is an example of mixed messages. In a family or social situation, such an event can result in great embarrassment and censure. On the other hand, among peers fart contests can be the source of great merriment. One situation is pulling in the anal sphincters and buttocks, the other is pushing out. (The other end of this, of course, is belching contests.) I am told by mothers that about the age of ten, boys go through a scatological phase where "shit" becomes a common word in their vocabulary.

This is a period of the beginning of misinformation about sex. Such information will generally pass from older boys to younger. These "facts" will be magnified in the imagination. A pattern of looking at sex grossly and crudely can emerge. Boys will play and identify with other boys. Boys who play with girls might be looked at with derision, including name-calling such as "sissy." Any sensitivity must not be displayed openly.

There is a lack of sensual touching for boys by both adult males and females, no doubt to avoid the fear of misinterpretation of intentions. In our more Puritanical culture, a male does not touch his genitals in public. One notable exception to this is the extreme sexual posturing, including genital touching, that frequently goes on at rock concerts, where presumably heterosexual musicians grope themselves to the delight of the fans.

In some of the Latin and Mediterranean cultures, men frequently grope their genitals in public. A conception that exists today in those countries is that men touch their sex to avert the evil eye and make a gesture of masculinity to invoke luck. In the past, did baseball pitchers grope their genitals for the same reason? This custom seems surprising and somewhat indecent for those of us from the more uptight northern cultures. One time I was in Puerto Rico with a friend from South America. We noticed how many men touched their genitals in public. We decided to mimic this gesture. My Brazilian friend had no problem since he had done this most of his life. I was totally unable to touch myself there in public. It was like an electric current pushing my hand away. So much for Midwest upbringing!

Until very recently, the showing of men's genitals pictorially was considered pornography. It is still considered as such by many. Years ago when I was directing a growth center in southern California, we sent out a brochure with a cover picture from a famous Leonardo da Vinci drawing of a man showing the male genitals. This was widely distributed. I received many calls from parents furious that their children would see such pornography. I expressed surprise that their children didn't know that male genitals existed.

It is not unusual for boys before puberty to become very modest. I have heard many fathers express surprise that where their sons had been very open about their bodies and had even taken showers with their father, they suddenly became very secretive about their genitals. Perhaps this is a normal phase. The child may have registered an unspoken message in the family or culture that the genitals and anus are "dirty." This also may be a message from their peers. This modesty seems to occur when boys become more interactive with each other. There is also the factor of how modest the parents are and their reaction to nudity.

One man can remember hot summer mornings when his naked father would come out of the bedroom on his way to the bathroom with his morning erection. His mother's response was "Cover that 'dirty' thing." This certainly set up a negative attitude about the erect penis. Since he still remembered this after many years, it obviously made an impression. Thirty years later he was visiting his parents after spending considerable time on the nude beaches of California. After he mentioned his total sun-tan, the talk of his parents and their friends turned very negative, includ-ing pornography among other things. He heard his mother say, "The body is dirty, dirty!" A "light bulb" came on in his mind explaining many of the problems he had experienced.

Such messages, verbal and nonverbal, establish confusing attitudes about the genitals and the anus. How can something that feels so plea-surable be regarded in such a negative fashion? This sets up a pattern that the feeling of pleasure is wrong. Perhaps, then, feelings in general are bad. One man who was born with a birth defect in his lower back (diagnosed many years later) loved to get a massage from his mother when he was young. After he was totally relaxed, she finished the massage with a hard slap to the buttocks which caused him to tense. The message seemed to be: "Don't enjoy yourself too much."

The unconscious method of shutting off feelings in the pelvis (or the body in general) is to block the breath into that area. The abdominal breath response will reach down as far as the middle abdomen, while the area of the pubic region will remain very quiet and unresponsive to the breath.

This habit no doubt starts in men as babies and is reinforced during growth and development stages. It can be accompanied by the tight anal canal and the pulling in of the penis.

Thus the stage is set for further confusions and misconceptions with the onset of hormones and the "terrible teens."

5

Puberty

WITH THE ADVENT OF SEXUAL MATURITY, the hormones stimulate a new set of emotional feelings. Since feelings in general are not considered manly, this can cause seemingly irrational behavior and confusion about one's self-identity. The voice change and the growth of body hair seem enough to deal with. Intensified pleasurable sexual urges in the genital (and possibly anal) region conflict with any previous message about that area being dirty, immoral, and repulsive, or other negative connotations. The first ejaculation may result in either surprised pleasure or revulsion and fear.

Recent studies have modified the concept of puberty. The responses described above may be the end of puberty rather than the beginning."Sex hormones" coming from the adrenal gland may be responsible for the behavioral hallmark of puberty, sexual attraction, as early as the age of six. Evidence indicates that "attraction" is far different from "action." There are several steps: attraction, actual desire, and finally a readiness to act on the desire. Thus, sexuality is a process of development rather than an event which emerges at a single moment in time.

Many psychotherapists assume that a man's sexual preference is established very young by which parent he felt attracted to. One man was asked the question by a new therapist. When the man said he had had sexual fantasies about both parents, the therapist refused to treat him.

Spontaneous erections, which can start very young, will elicit feelings of delight in private and embarrassment in public. The feelings of guilt become more intense. Most men have memories of embarrassing erections. One was the erotic effect of the vibrations sitting on a bus; when he reached his stop and had to get up, he tried to cover his erection as best he could with books or clothing. There are many stories of hard-ons in school and the contortions to cover at the end of the class. Since nudity is considered pornography in some families, observing nude statues can result in arousal of the penis. The combination of feelings of pleasure and embarrassment will result in thoughts that pleasure is embarrassing. The need for control continues the unconscious efforts to block feelings in the genitals.

Ejaculation is a new toy and a wonder. Wet dreams are humiliating when the evidence is found. Masturbation, which often starts at a younger age as play, now has a startling endpoint. Orgasms give rise to new sensations. In many families, masturbation is not discussed, and intuitively the boy knows that this process is considered unhealthy, improper, and immoral. It is something that must be done in great secrecy and often rapidly to avoid discovery. The feeling of guilt is a frequent companion. The sensuous feelings that accompany the buildup to orgasm and ejaculation are not allowed when speed is required.

A man told me that when he was in his teens, he would masturbate while sitting on the toilet stool so the ejaculate could go directly into the toilet. If he took too long, his mother would pound on the bathroom door."What's taking you so long? You're not playing with yourself, are you?" So he knew that speed was of the essence. This begins the habitual pattern of "getting off" as quickly as possible when an erection occurs.

A pattern is established whereby the prolonged pleasure of foreplay will be difficult if not impossible in future sexual activity. Many women (and gay men) complain that their partner comes quickly and then either rolls over to sleep or puts on his pants and goes home. This pattern starts early. It also triggers the pattern of isolating the pleasure of the orgasm to the penis—there is no time to feel the effects in the rest of the body.

As mentioned earlier, circumcision was initially introduced in this country as a cure for masturbation. The negative feelings about the natural process of masturbation continue to this day. I can remember in the

'40s, boys were teasing about jerking-off causing blindness, insanity, and the growing of hair on the palms of your hands. Many of us tentatively checked daily for any hair growth on our palms. In a Rolfing class, a practitioner had been burned on his palms and had had skin transplants from other parts of his body. As a result, he had hair on his palms. One of the older practitioners spoke up, "That will teach you to play with that thing!" It caused much hilarity in the class and we all knew what he was talking about.

It is at this phase of development that boys begin to tell lies. These lies are mostly about sex. In addition to the secrecy about masturbation, this is also the period of the start of sexual experimentation. Early on, this will frequently involve other boys. Comparisons of the size of the penis and the amount of pubic and facial hair can be direct or overt. Some of the more adventuresome may be involved in "circle-jerks." There may be some jovial or rough grabbing of the genitals and/or the buttocks but no intimate or sensual touching. Peer pressure is not to talk about sexual feelings. The possibilities are either no talk or accusatory comments or ridicule.

From both peers and family there is a lack of any reinforcement about "feeling good" about the genitals and the anus—or the body in general. The body (the pelvic area especially) is not talked about sympathetically. In many families, the focus is completely on the development of the mind, not the body. Any physical consideration involves the development of the external body—becoming more muscular like a man. Generally no education or information about internal subtle movements or emotions is desired.

The age at which the boy reaches sexual maturity will be a factor in how the boy handles this development. The majority of boys will reach maturity as indicated by pubic and facial hair and genital development later in their teens. A lower percentage develop the physical characteristics as early as twelve years of age. Either case can create a shyness in school showers or at urinals. Those who reach physical maturity early may feel pride in their development and yet can be a subject of jokes and teasing by peers. Conversely, those who develop late in their teens can feel inadequate, may worry if they will ever catch up physically, and can be a subject of derision. The focus on the penis size and erection ability as a measure of manhood becomes established.

The concerns about sexual orientation become stronger at this time. It is generally agreed that many boys relate sexually in some way to other boys during this period. Often a desire for physical contact will be accomplished through contact sports or rough-housing on the playground or in the showers. There is nonverbal agreement that there is nothing abnormal in slapping a butt, hugging as a group, wrestling, or even a sport pileup. The contact is there and it is in no way sensual. This is seen all the time in adult sports. Whatever feelings are elicited by this contact are buried. More sensitive touching may occur, such as a pat on the back or roughly stroking the hair. The more sensitive or non-athletic boy will generally have more of a problem about touching and being touched. The relation of touching only for sex becomes more firmly established.

Many boys will practice sex play with other boys which focuses on the penis. This is considered a phase. Gay men can find that it is a phase that doesn't end. Many will push their feelings aside and "act" the straight life for many years. Whether gay or straight, the confusion about the interaction of emotions, touching, and sex is more pronounced at this period of development. This reinforces the inhibition of body sensitivity and the blocking of internal physical and emotional awareness.

6

Genital Development

BEFORE CONSIDERING HOW the early structural and emotional development manifests itself in adult structure and function, it seems appropriate to discuss the development of the male reproductive system. (The majority of men are totally ignorant about how their genitals are put together and most of them prefer to stay that way.) The penis and the testicles develop independently. It is only late in fetal development that they become positioned adjacent to each other. In early development, the penis and the anus are more closely interrelated than the penis and the testicles.

The testicles: The first indication of primitive testes occurs adjacent to the primitive kidney (mesonephros) in the chest region about the end of the first month of pregnancy. The majority of this primitive kidney degenerates as the adult kidney (metanephros) develops lower in the abdominal cavity. The ducts of the primitive kidney remain as the duct system for the testes after the remainder of the kidney has disappeared (Fig. 6-1).

As development occurs, the body of the fetus becomes larger and longer. The testes are connected to the floor of the primitive pelvis by a ligament (gubernaculum testis). This ligament is not elastic and as the body as a whole elongates, the testes are "pulled down" by the rigidity of the ligament. (Note: The ovaries also "descend" into the abdominal region.) The ligament actually shortens later, guiding the testis through

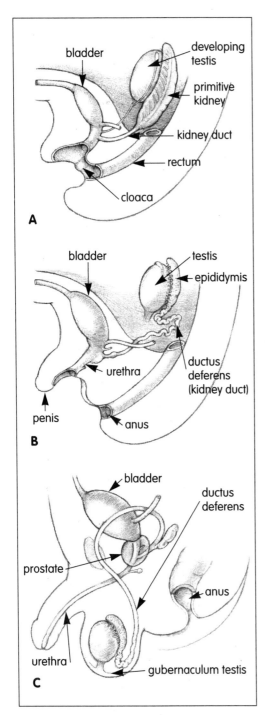

A

- bladder
- developing testis
- primitive kidney
- kidney duct
- rectum
- cloaca

B

- bladder
- testis
- epididymis
- urethra
- ductus deferens (kidney duct)
- penis
- anus

C

- bladder
- ductus deferens
- prostate
- anus
- urethra
- gubernaculum testis

the inguinal canal, over the pubic bone, and down into the scrotal swellings. The scrotal swellings lie on either side of the developing penis (Fig. 3-1). The inguinal canal is formed by the fusion of the abdominal oblique muscles in the lower abdomen to form a type of sling. The lower boundary of these abdominal muscles is termed the inguinal ligament, with the inguinal canal above it. At the time of the testicle descent through the inguinal canal—about the seventh or eighth month of pregnancy—the abdominal muscles consist mainly of thin, transparent fascia layers. The testicles therefore leave the security of the body cavity to become more externally exposed. I have previously suggested that this could initiate castration fears in the mid-groin region (Fig. 6-2).

Normally the inguinal canal closes after the testis migrates through it. It contains the spermatic cord, which is composed of the blood vessels and nerves of the testes plus the ductus deferens, the duct carrying the sperm from the testicles to the penis. The ductus deferens is the remnant of the primitive kidney. In some men, this canal re-

---

◄ FIGURE 6-1

Development of the male reproductive system

(A) Development of the testes in relation to the primitive kidney; (B) degeneration of the kidney with the duct system remaining; (C) descent of the testes into the scrotum.

mains open throughout life and the testes can rise up into the canal, especially at the time of arousal. This is not a problem unless they get stuck there.

The penis: In lower vertebrates, there is a common posterior chamber into which fecal, urinary, and reproductive products all pass, and from which they are expelled to the exterior. This is called a cloaca. In humans, as well as other mammals, the cloaca is present in early stages of development and is subdivided in the second month of pregnancy. The initial divisions are a dorsal (back) rectum and a ventral (front) bladder and urogenital sinus. This division is accomplished by a horizontal fold called the urorectal septum (Fig. 6-3). An analogy would be the curtain in a theater which divides the stage from the auditorium when it is lowered.

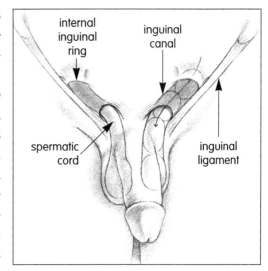

FIGURE 6-2
Pathway of descent of testicles prior to birth
Internal inguinal ring is exit point of testicle from abdominal cavity.

The septum or fold extends down to the outer membrane at the end of the primitive digestive tract, the cloacal membrane. The septum projects out from the surface, forming the perineal body and separating the anal opening from that of the urogenital sinus. The opening of the urogenital sinus lies at the base of the phallus. The phallus is a projection which occurs in the second month of pregnancy and begins its development into the penis under the influence of fetal androgens (male hormones). The fetal androgens are present by the second month of pregnancy and also determine the differentiation of the testes.

In the female, the phallus forms the clitoris. In the male, the phallus elongates with a groove on the underside. This groove is continuous with the opening of the urogenital sinus. The groove ultimately extends to the end of the penis. The sides of the groove will fuse to form a tube. This fusion takes place all the way to the anus. The "scar" from this fusion is evident in the adult on the underside of the penis, dividing the scrotum

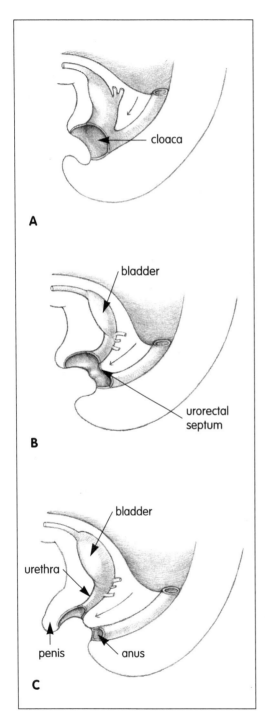

A

B

C

cloaca

bladder

urorectal
septum

bladder

urethra

penis   anus

into two halves, and up to the anus (Fig. 6-2). In some men, the fusion is not complete to the end of the penis. This is a condition called hypospadias. It is not a problem if it causes the opening of the penis to extend down only into the base of the glans (head) of the penis. Otherwise, surgical intervention is necessary. As a side note, a boy with hypospadias should not be circumcised.

The urogenital sinus becomes the bladder and the prostatic urethra. The prostate has arisen as glandular outgrowths from the urethra at the base of the bladder. The ductus deferens (spermatic duct) travels from the testes in the scrotum through the inguinal canal, and loops medially to connect to the prostatic urethra (Fig. 6-1).

Thus the testicles and the penis, which are grouped together as genitals, arise from very different origins.

◄ FIGURE 6-3
**Separation of urogenital sinus and bladder
from anal canal**
Development from fifth (A) to eighth
(C) week of pregnancy.

7

Genital Structure

T HE PENIS IS OFTEN CONSIDERED as a separate entity from the rest of the body, sometimes with its own life and a name. But of course the penis is very much a part of the whole body; it is not autonomous. The penis is under the control of the nervous system—a combination of voluntary and involuntary innervations. By examining the structure of the genitals in detail, we can better understand the interactions by which men protect them.

The penis consists of a root located in the perineum (the area between the legs that we sit on; in women it contains the vaginal opening) and a free, normally pendulous portion, termed the corpus or body, which is completely enveloped in skin. It consists of three bodies of erectile tissue which extend through most of the length of the penis. The upper two bodies, the corpora cavernosa, consist of highly vascular connective tissue or fascia. They are firmly attached to the margins of the arch of the pubic bone. They do not extend to the end of the penis. The lower body, the corpus spongiosum, contains—in addition to the vascular fascia—the penile urethra or duct coming from the prostatic urethra. The glans or head of the penis is the expansion at the end of the corpus spongiosum. The base of the corpus spongiosum is firmly attached to the fascia of the perineum or urogenital diaphragm (Fig. 7-1).

Erection is controlled by the autonomic nervous system affecting the blood vessels of the penis. The parasympathetic fibers (the relaxing part

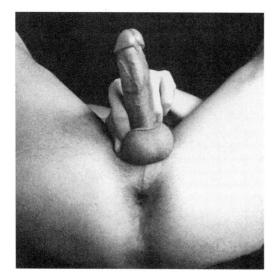 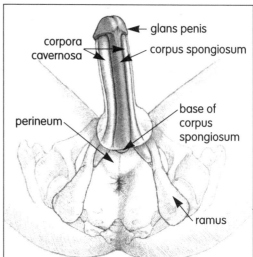

FIGURE 7-1
Structure of the penis

of the involuntary nervous system) in the nerves of the corpora cause a dilation of the small arteries. This dilation increases blood flow into the blood sinuses, resulting in a distension of all three corpora. This increased volume of blood applies pressure to the veins leading from the sinuses and decreases the venous flow from the tissue. After ejaculation or time and lack of energy, it is assumed that the sympathetic fibers or involuntary stimulating nerves constrict the arteries, reducing the blood flow into the sinuses and allowing the blood to flow back into the veins. The penis can then return to its flaccid state.

It has been assumed that the dorsal veins which lie on top of the corpora cavernosa are the major venous factor in erection. Over the years I have observed that there are veins on the sides of the penis which also serve in that function. In many cases pressure on the left side of the base of the penis will produce an erection. Pressing on this side can also help increase the rigidity of the erection during sexual activity.

The penis is often referred to as a "muscle." There is no muscle in the penis itself except for the smooth muscle of the blood vessels. There are muscles that can be considered extensions of the perineum which are

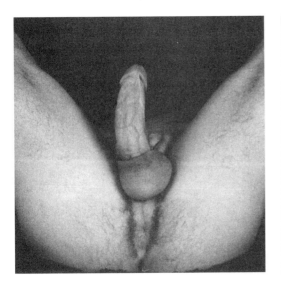
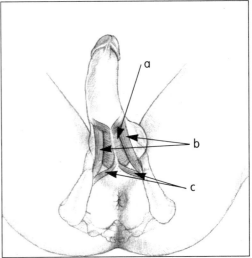

FIGURE 7-2
Muscles of the penis
(a) bulbospongiosus m. (b) ischiocavernosa m. (c) transverse perineal m.

located at the base of the penis. The bulbospongiosus arises from the perineal body and extends in a Y-shape around the base of the corpus spongiosum. The muscle aids in the emptying of the urethra, after the bladder has expelled its contents, the final spurts. It can be used to stop the flow of urine. There may be some contribution to erection.

The ischiocavernosa is a pair of muscles that covers the base of the corpora cavernosa. They arise from the V-shaped ramus of the ischial bone, extending back to the ischial tuberosities, the "sitz" bones (Fig. 7-2). These muscles may play a more specific part in maintaining erection of the penis. With palpation, it often feels as though these muscles become glued to the bony rami, resembling the texture of beef jerky. This lack of tone will make them relatively non-functional.

The perineum or urogenital diaphragm fills the area between the ischial rami (the bony platform we sit on). Midway between the tuberosities at the end of the rami is the perineal body. This is a fibromuscular node with fascial and muscular attachments in front to the bulbospongiosus of the penis and behind to the external sphincter of the anus. It also receives

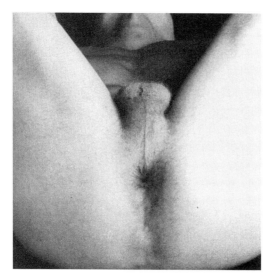 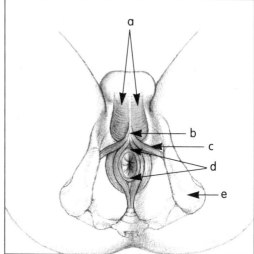

FIGURE 7-3
Muscular connections in the perineal region
(a) bulbospongiosus m. (b) perineal body (c) transverse perineal muscles
(d) external anal sphincter (e) ischial tuberosity

fibers from the transverse perineal muscles which make up most of the perineum, and from the levator ani or pelvic diaphragm (Figs. 7-3).

The perineal body, therefore, serves as an interface between the anus and the penis. Habitual contraction or flaccidity of the area will affect its structure and function. Constant tightness would pull the anus and penis into the body, resulting in constipation or difficulty in initiating urination. Lack of tone of the muscle and fascia could lead to incontinence for urine and/or feces.

The levator ani or pelvic diaphragm (deep to the perineum) extends from the inner surface of the pubic bone to the coccyx. It has some connection to part of the external anal sphincter, to the perineal body, and possibly to the base of the bulbospongiosus. This is referred to as the floor of the pelvis (Fig. 7-4). This is the bottom of the abdominal cavity. Potentially, the so-called "abdominal breathing" can be felt this far down.

In front, there are two ligaments that suspend the penis. One, the fundiform ligament, arises from the linea alba (midline) of the sheath of the

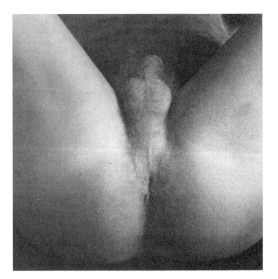
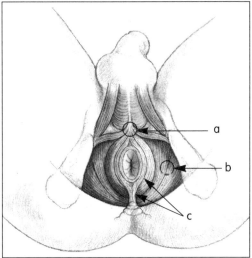

FIGURE 7-4
Pelvic and urogenital diaphragms
(a) urogenital diaphragm (perineum) (b) pelvic diaphragm (levator ani)
(c) external anal sphincter

rectus abdominus and wraps around the penis in a sling-like arrangement. The suspensory ligament arises from the pubic symphysis and also wraps around the penis (Fig. 7-5). Tightening of the abdominal muscles by sit-ups and other exercises is often considered a cosmetic need in our culture. This can create a shortening of the abdominal muscles between the pubic bone and the umbilicus (belly button) where the muscle and fascia have become habitually tense. Since the suspending ligaments are a continuation of the rectus abdominal fascia, such tightness will result in a constant pull upward and inward of the penis. This can lead to a deadening of the feeling in the penis, especially since the breath response will not reach that region.

It is estimated that one to three inches of the penis may be internal, sometimes buried in the layer of fatty tissue over the pubic bone. The penis is not a muscle—it cannot be "pumped up" like the skeletal muscles of the body. It may become smaller with lack of use. The length of external penis may be determined by the flaccidness or rigidity of the

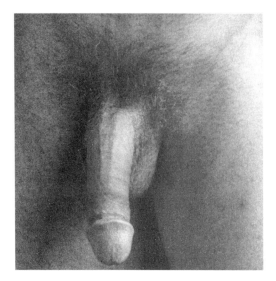
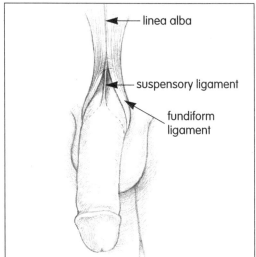

FIGURE 7-5
Suspending ligaments of the penis

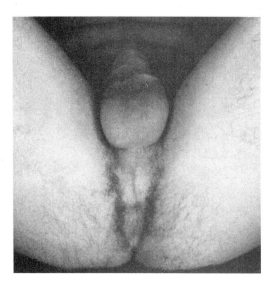
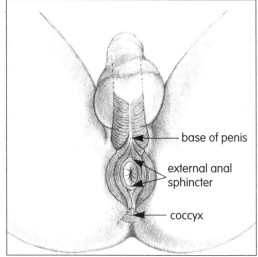

FIGURE 7-6
Muscular connection of the penis to the coccyx (tailbone)

muscles behind and above the penis. The tone of the abdominal muscles will determine the lift of the suspending ligaments. The tone of the mus-

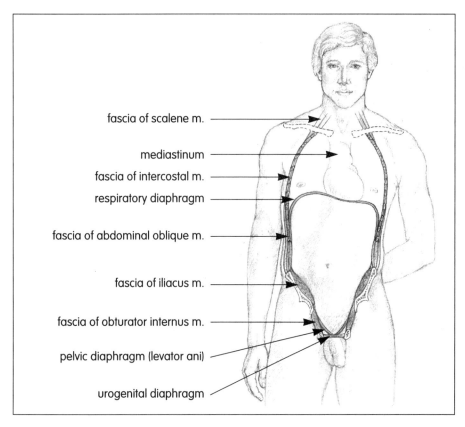

fascia of scalene m.

mediastinum

fascia of intercostal m.

respiratory diaphragm

fascia of abdominal oblique m.

fascia of iliacus m.

fascia of obturator internus m.

pelvic diaphragm (levator ani)

urogenital diaphragm

FIGURE 7-7
Diaphragms of the body cavity

cles of the perineum (urogenital diaphragm) and/or the pelvic diaphragm (levator ani) may cause a pulling in of the base of the penis. A tight anus will pull on the base of the penis through the connection of the external sphincter with the perineal body (Fig. 7-6). Any or all of these conditions translate into a loss of feeling and a problem with function.

Fascial connections from both the pelvic and urogenital diaphragms will extend to the fascia of the obturator internus muscle, from there to the fascia of the iliacus muscle, to the fascia of the abdominal oblique muscles, and to the fascia of the respiratory diaphragm. The genital area does not exist in isolation (Fig. 7-7). A lack of elasticity of the diaphragms will affect the tissues above and vice versa.

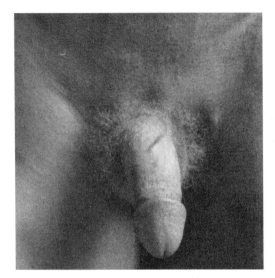 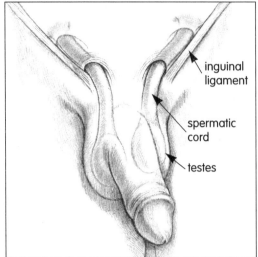

FIGURE 7-8
Male genitals

The **testicles** lie on either side of and slightly behind the penis. They are located in the scrotal sac, the skin of which is continuous with the skin of the penis. Each testicle is suspended by a spermatic cord which contains the blood and nerve supply of the testes and the spermatic duct (ductus deferens). The cord crosses the pubic bone and enters the external opening of the inguinal canal. It continues diagonally upward through the inguinal canal to the internal opening into the body cavity. From there the spermatic duct angles down to enter the prostatic urethra at the base of the bladder (Fig. 7-8).

The internal opening or internal ring of the inguinal canal is the site of inguinal hernias. These seem to be related to tightness in the surrounding musculature and fascia. The internal ring can be considered a "weak" area. It is formed by an opening in the tendonous extensions of the abdominal oblique muscles with no supporting muscle involved. Tightness in the psoas and the abdominals will pull the tissue apart, enlarging the opening so that a loop of the gut can slip through and become "herniated." The symptoms of incipient hernia have often been relieved by reducing the tightness of the surrounding musculature, thereby reducing the pull on the internal ring.

The **scrotal sac** is divided into two compartments by a septum. On the surface one can see the "scar" or raphe continuous with that of the underside of the penis. This indicates the dual origin of the scrotum. Generally the left testicle hangs lower than the right. It has been speculated that this occurs because the left side descends first before birth. Also, the spermatic cord frequently adheres tightly to the side of the penis on the left causing the penis to point to the left. It has been estimated that 75% of men hang to the left (Fig. 7-9).

The wall of the scrotum contains the dartos muscle. This is the extension of the subcutaneous fascia of the abdominal wall and may be an extension of the external abdominal oblique muscle. This is non-skeletal muscle, responding to involuntary control. It causes the folds of the scrotum and will respond to stimuli such as cold or sexual arousal by shrinking up to the body wall. The cremaster muscle seems to be the muscle of the spermatic cord. Its contraction will draw the testes up to the body. There seem to be two mechanisms in the involuntary response to cold and other stimuli—one compressing the scrotal wall and the other raising the testicles. Generally they will act together, but they can act individually. There is a "cremaster reflex" on the inner thigh. When that area is stimulated by light touching, the testicle on that side will be drawn up by the cremaster muscle. The dartos muscle is not affected by this reflex. Sexual arousal will generally cause the testicles to be pulled up to the body and the scrotal sac will tighten, forming many folds in the wall (Fig. 7-10).

Since normal body temperature is too warm for proper sperm production, the function of the scrotal muscles is to aid in the regulation of the temperature of the testicles. When it is hot, the testicles will hang loose, allowing for cooling away from the body proper. In the cold, the testicles are drawn up close to the body for warmth. Studies in England have shown that men who consistently wear tight briefs have a lower sperm production than those men who wear looser underwear. Today when a man has a fertility problem, it is common for the doctor to recommend boxer-type shorts.

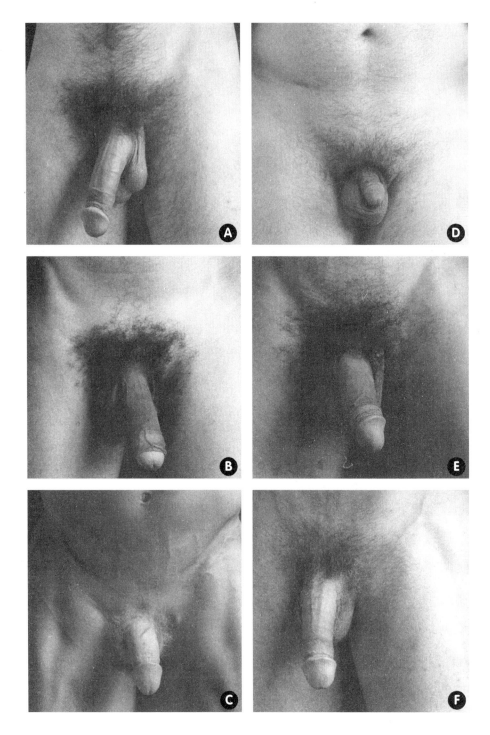

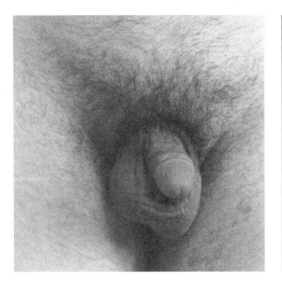
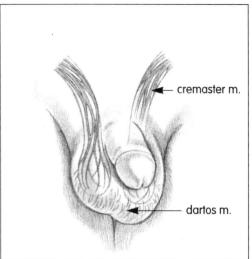

— cremaster m.

— dartos m.

FIGURE 7-10
Muscles of the scrotum

The penis does not exist in isolation. Its fascia is continuous with that of the perineum, the rectus abdominus muscle, and the adductor muscles of the inner thigh. This was demonstrated in a water skiing accident that happened to a friend of mine. The skis were pointed outward when he started off. He held on to the rope, attempting to bring the skis together. His legs spread further and further apart until he felt a "snap" in his groin area. Too late, he let go of the rope. The results were not only stiffness in the upper leg muscles and difficulty sitting down (especially on the toilet), but also a large, purplish haematoma over the pubic bone area which extended into the shaft of the penis. Such results of a pull on the inner adductor muscles affecting the penis can be explained by fascial continuity.

◄ FIGURE 7-9
Variations of penis
Note that one of the six (A) hangs to the right, and one of the six (B) is uncircumcised. Chosen randomly, the models above roughly approximate the normal variations in the U.S. Size variation is also apparent.

8

Anus

T HE USUAL CONCEPT of "tight ass" is habitually tensed external muscle. The gluteus maximus is the most external and the largest muscle of the buttocks. It extends diagonally from the back of the crest of the pelvic bone (ilium), across the ischial tuberosities, and continues down the side of the thigh via the iliotibial tract (Fig. 8-1). It is frequently

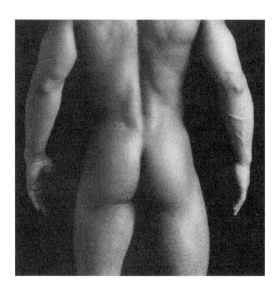 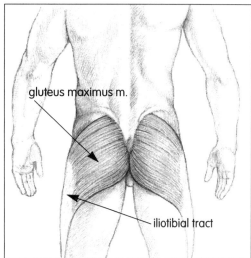

FIGURE 8-1
Gluteus maximus and attachments

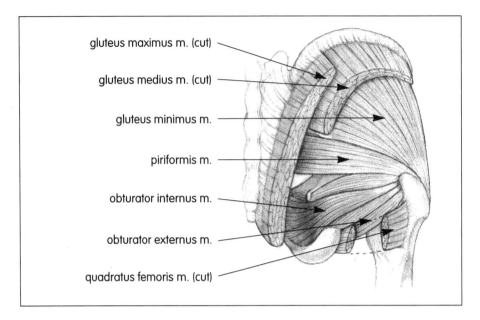

FIGURE 8-2
"Lateral" rotators of the thigh

held in a partially contracted condition, affecting the muscles and fascia
of the lower back and the hamstrings. Its contraction in walking is related
to turned-out feet and legs—the "duck walk." Dancers often pride themselves on walking in a permanent turnout.

Under the gluteus maximus is a group of short muscles which are
termed the external or lateral rotators. These muscles are the piriformis,
the obturator internus and externus, the superior and inferior gamelli,
the quadratus femoris, and the gluteus minimus. Although the latter is
not usually included in this group, it seems logical to do so since it is the
uppermost muscle in the fan-like arrangement of the rotators behind the
femur. Although each muscle arises from a different part of the ilium, they
attach more or less in a row to the back part of the trochanter (bony projection) of the femur (Fig. 8-2).

The method of external protection of the anal area varies. In men with
very hard, solid-textured, often rounded butts, the gluteus maximus is
like iron. The cheeks are very tightly held together. Since the normal angle

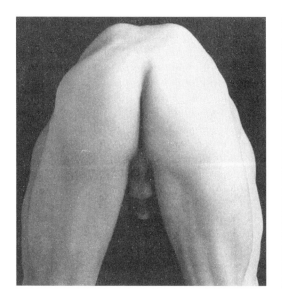 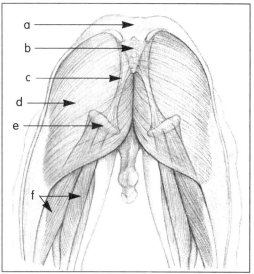

FIGURE 8-3
Folding of gluteus maximus around sacrotubrous ligament
(a) sacrum (b) coccyx (c) sacrotubrous ligament (d) gluteus maximus m.
(e) ischial tuberosity (f) hamstring m.

of the pull of the maximus is diagonal across the pelvis from the sacrum
to the iliotibial tract on the outside of the thigh, its habitual pull would
draw the femur back up the pelvis at an oblique angle—back and
upwards. This does not explain the tightness of the cleft. The very lowest segment of the gluteus maximus has its upper attachment to the coccyx (tailbone). This lowest part will fold inward, around the tough
sacrotubrous ligament, which extends from the lower sacrum to the ischial
tuberosities (Fig. 8-3). This lower section of the gluteus maximus muscle
crosses the tuberosities. If this part of the maximus is pulled tight, it will
fold more around the ligament, pulling the cheeks closer together. It will
also bring the tuberosities closer together. Thus the cleft or space between
the muscles becomes a tight slit, almost impenetrable by hand. The coccyx is very deep (Fig. 8-4). This type of buttocks is often seen in heavy
body builders, football players, and wrestlers. There is no doubt a genetic

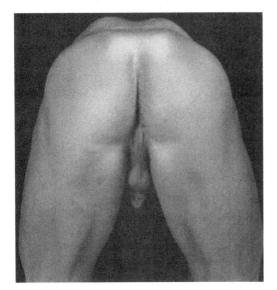 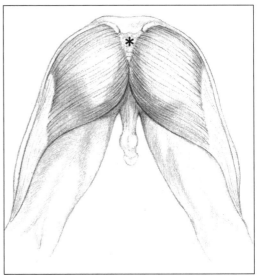

FIGURE 8-4
(*) Deep coccyx in body builder

aspect to the type of muscle, which may indicate why these men became involved in these athletic activities.

In men with spongy to soft cheeks, the gluteus maximus is underused and the rotators will become overly tight in compensation. They can feel like steel cables under the softer gluteus maximus. This will bring the greater trochanter of the femur directly back, restricting the movement in the joint. It will create a dimple on the side of the buttocks which unfortunately is considered sexy by many. In this case, it is very difficult to feel any space between the back of the femur and the bony pelvis. The coccyx is close to the surface and usually easy to palpate.

Any combination of chronically tense pelvic muscles locks the hip joint. It is very common for men not to use the hip joint in walking. The movement comes from the lower back, bypassing the hip joint, and creating a stiff gait. This movement habit may start early to avoid swinging the hips, which many a man fears will cause confusion about his sexual orientation.

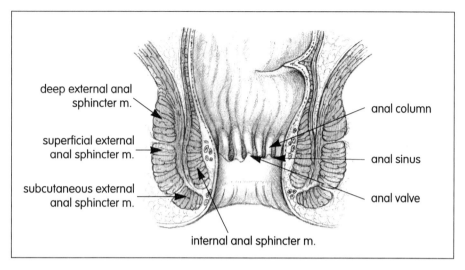

deep external anal
sphincter m.

superficial external
anal sphincter m.

subcutaneous external
anal sphincter m.

anal column

anal sinus

anal valve

internal anal sphincter m.

FIGURE 8-5
Anal sphincters

The internal components of this protection are the sphincter muscles of the anus which form the anal canal. Since these appear to be isolated in the fatty tissue of the ischio-rectal fossa, their connection to the rest of the pelvic structure is not immediately apparent. A more detailed examination reveals the connections between the anal sphincters and other structures of the pelvis, including the male genitalia. These connections clarify how a habitually tense or contracted anus will affect the entire pelvis, and thus the structure of the entire body.

The anal canal consists of an external sphincter with three layers and an internal sphincter (Fig. 8-5). The internal sphincter is a mucous membrane continuous with the rectum, the lowest part of the large intestine. The epithelium is a simple columnar layer composed of columnar absorbing cells. The muscle layers are circular smooth (involuntary) muscle. The nervous innervation is the sympathetic and parasympathetic (autonomic) nervous system. This part of the anal canal is less sensitive to touch and very sensitive to pressure.

The mucous membrane of the internal sphincter is raised by rectal veins to a number of vertical anal columns. The depressions between are referred to as the anal sinuses. These columns terminate at the anal valves, which indicate the separation between the internal and external sphincters (Fig. 8-5). The rectal veins may form hemorrhoids in the anal columns. At defecation the entire mucous membrane may be extruded in front of the fecal mass, including the hemorrhoid area. The lower part of the anal canal is opened and flattened, so that the mucous membrane of the upper part appears at the surface.

Normally the length of the anal wall will be returned to its closed state by the muscle tone of the external sphincter. If the rectal veins remain dilated, the hemorrhoids or varicosities may remain external. These can sometimes be replaced manually. If the hemorrhoids are severe, surgery is necessary. Following such surgery, there will be much discomfort and sensitivity. Dietary care must be taken to keep the bowels softer. This results in a more intense negative attitude about the anus.

Since the internal sphincter is controlled by the autonomic nervous system, it normally functions reflexively. The rectal reflex, caused by the pressure of feces, involves the automatic relaxation of the internal sphincter and a partial draining of the blood from the anal columns. If this reflex is ignored, as is often taught in toilet training, the reflex fades and the internal sphincter stops relaxing. The result is the need for pushing and straining in bowel movements, eventually raising the possibility of hemorrhoids, bleeding, or other injury to the anal canal. The reflex can be retrained by breathing and relaxation.

The surface covering (epithelium) of the external sphincter is continuous with the epidermis of the skin, which is called stratified squamous. The surface of this epithelium is not cornified (keratinized or horny), and near the anal orifice it contains hairs, sweat glands, sebaceous glands, and tactile nerve endings like the skin. The underlying muscle layers are skeletal (voluntary) muscle with nerve innervation from branches of the fourth sacral nerve. The layers of the external sphincter are classified as subcutaneous, superficial, and deep. The skeletal muscle layers are under the control of "will" and usually in a state of tonic contraction (tight ass)!

An over-simplification of the above would be that the external sphincter is controlled by the conscious and the internal by the unconscious.

The subcutaneous part of the external sphincter consists of horizontal

fibers which surround the lowest part of
the anal canal. It extends from below the
lower borders of the internal anal sphincter down to just below the skin. A few of
the muscle fibers attach to the perineal
body in front and to the anococcygeal ligament behind.

The superficial part lies below the subcutaneous part and is elliptical in shape.
The muscles attach to the coccyx by the
anococcygeal ligament and to the central
tendon of the perineum, which is termed
the perineal body (Fig. 8-6).

The perineum lies at the bottom of the
pelvis between the legs. It consists of two
triangular areas, one of which is the posterior part in front of the coccyx containing the anus and anal sphincters. In front,
between the V-shaped bony rami, is a
muscular and fascial layer termed the urogenital diaphragm or urogenital triangle.
The perineal body or central tendon lies

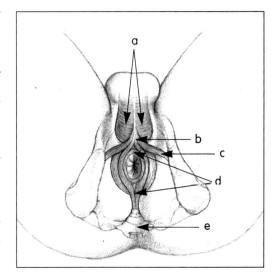

FIGURE 8-6
**Muscular connections
in the perineal region**
(a)bulbospongiosus m. of the penis
(b) perineal body (c) transverse perineal
muscles (d) external anal sphincter
(e) coccyx

in the medial plane of this triangle. The muscles that converge and inter-
lace into this body are: the external anal sphincter, the muscles that support the base of the penis (bulbospongiosus), and four muscles that form
the body of the diaphragm (the perineal muscles) (Fig. 8-6).

One of my clients referred to the perineum as the "t'aint" region."T'aint
your anus and t'aint your balls." Other clients have called it "the dirty
region." I have wondered if these negative comments may not be related
to the fact that this is the location of the vagina in women. Men may not
want to consider anything in their bodies to be similar to a part of a
woman's body.

The connection by the external anal sphincter of the coccyx to the base
of the penis clarifies how habitual contraction of the anal sphincter will
draw the penis closer to the coccyx, and over time of development will

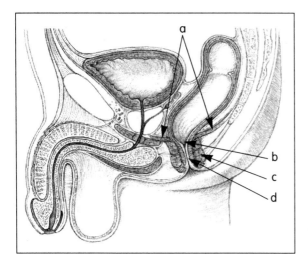

FIGURE 8-7

Saggital view of male pelvis

(a) levator ani (pelvic diaphragm) (b) area of anorectal ring of muscle (c) deep external anal sphincter (d) internal anal sphincter

contract and reduce the size of the perineum (Figs. 8-6, 8-7). Visualize the perineum like a fan with the perineal body (central tendon) at the base and the outer edges connecting to the inverted V-shaped bony rami. The drawing back of the perineal body at the base by the sphincter muscle would narrow the perineum and bring the bones of the rami closer together. This would impede the circulation to the tissues of the perineum. As a result, the space between the rami would be narrow and barely palpable and the tissue texture would be toughened. This is the case in many men, where the space between the rami is barely palpable and the tissue between feels like cement.

The toughness or lack of tone of the tissue between the rami would correlate with a lack of feeling in the perineum and a lack of breath to the area. It would interfere with easy pelvic movement and sexual enjoyment. Since the male pelvis is already more narrow than the female, the tightness of the tissue would intensify the narrowness of the structure. The hamstrings on the back of the legs, which more or less arise from the ischial tuberosities, would be rotated toward each other (Fig. 8-8). Thus the movement between the pelvis and legs would become even more restricted.

The deep, internal part of the external sphincter is a thick annular band. This is at the level where the rectum penetrates the levator ani (the pelvic diaphragm) and becomes the anal canal. Some of the fibers of the levator ani form a sling around the upper anal canal coming from the pelvic side to the pubic bone, the puborectalis. There are also fibers from this part which connect to the anococcygeal ligament. An anorectal ring of muscle is formed by the puborectalis, the deep external sphincter, and the internal sphincter (Fig 8-7). This ring aids in rectal continence and thus serves as a supplement to the sphincters.

These muscular interactions and connections demonstrate how the habitual contraction of the anal sphincter muscles, especially at an early age, will affect the ease or dis-ease of function of the genitals, the diaphragms of the pelvis, and the lower digestive tract. A much broader effect can be envisioned if one considers the fascial connections. Since muscles start and stop, the fascial continuations allow for a larger dimension of potential effects.

The fascia of the external sphincter will be continuous with that of the urogenital diaphragm (perineum) and with the muscles of the penis as well as with the fascia of the penis itself (the penis being primarily vascularized fascia). At the margins of the diaphragm, the fascia is continuous below with that of the adductors of the thigh. Above, the fascia is continuous with that of the obturator internus, the pelvic diaphragm (levator ani), the iliacus, the internal abdominal obliques, and up to the res-

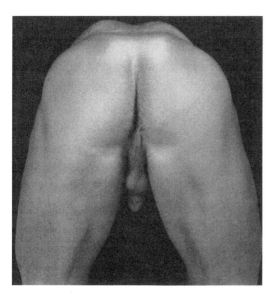
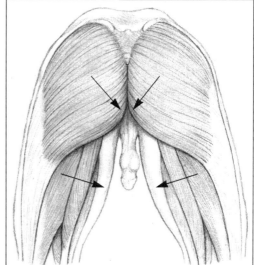

FIGURE 8-8
Tight ass and hamstrings
Arrows indicate direction of muscle movement.

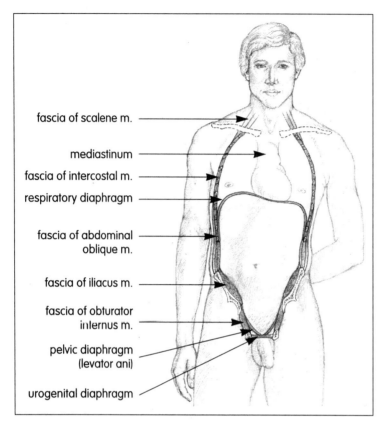

fascia of scalene m. ———————

mediastinum ———————

fascia of intercostal m. ———————

respiratory diaphragm ———————

fascia of abdominal —————
oblique m.

fascia of iliacus m. ———————

fascia of obturator
internus m. ———————

pelvic diaphragm ———————
(levator ani)

urogenital diaphragm ———————

FIGURE 8-9
Body diaphragms

piratory diaphragm (Fig. 8-9).

Thus with the habitual tightening of the anal sphincters and the subsequent pulling in of the penis, we can visualize the pulling down of the lower body trunk and the interference with breathing. On a local level, the lack of ability to relax these muscles can lead to constipation, hemorrhoids, and anal tears.

Since the anus is one of the chronic centers of tension, it is difficult to think of it as elastic. However, its flexibility has been demonstrated by its ability to accommodate by relaxation the insertion of finger or fingers, of dildos of various sizes, of the penis in anal sex, and of a hand without apparent damage. The latter is usually facilitated with a mixture of intoxicants (drugs and/or alcohol), fantasy, foreplay, and the learned ability to mix passion and relaxation. Having worked with individuals who engaged in these activities, I was surprised to find that under everyday circumstances their anal sphincters were as tight as anyone else's.

9

Erections

SOME YEARS AGO at the regional Rolfing meeting, a number of the women Rolfers complained about their male clients getting erections during the work. They were indignant that the client was having sexual feelings toward them when they had done nothing to cause this. A visiting male Rolfing teacher, in a very macho way, indicated that this was a problem only for women Rolfers; they should discuss it with each other. This meant, of course, that it had never happened to him. I pointed out that the erections were a sign of relaxation of the man's body and had nothing to do with them personally. The women were then even more indignant! They apparently didn't like the implication that they had no sex appeal.

The male Rolfing teacher was no doubt too uptight to work extensively in the male pelvis. My procedure at that time was to turn out the light at the end of a session on the pelvis and leave the client to enjoy his sensations by himself. At the time I left the room, there was no sign of arousal. When I returned I was often startled to find the client relaxed with a full erection. The usual comment was: "I've never felt so relaxed in my life." There was no comment or embarrassment about the state of his penis. It seemed that he was not even aware of the situation.

My wonder was, "Erection ... relaxation?" This did not coincide with my understanding of erections. I had been raised with the nonverbal cultural and verbal peer messages that erection happened only when a man was "hot to trot" sexually and MUST be followed by sexual activity or masturbation. Under any other circumstance, it was improper and crude. Could there be another circumstance for this condition?

I began to consider that there can be at least two types of erections. One is a result of erotic stimulation and another is associated with relaxation and sensual feelings about yourself. It has been estimated that men have several erections during sleep which have nothing to do with the need to urinate. (The pressure of a full bladder can also cause an erection.) The erections are not necessarily associated with erotic dreams. It just feels good. I have been told by several younger men that the morning erection is not necessarily a "piss hard-on." It often can be related to more erotic feelings, while some of those in the middle of the night are not.

Nowadays when a man gets aroused during a Rolfing session and is aware of it, he may ask about its significance. I ask, "Doesn't it feel good?" The usual response is something like, "Oh, yes." I tell them to just enjoy the feeling. These erections are not lasting. I usually mention that when a man gets older, erections don't happen as often and that when one does happen, its occurrence gives a feeling of pleasure. I also say that I don't take their condition personally, which puts humor into the situation.

As I mentioned, some men are so insensitive to their bodily sensations that they are not aware of having an erection when relaxed. It could be that their awareness of their body happens only when the sexual feelings are high. Even in that case, the feeling is often only in the penis, not in the rest of the body.

An unfortunate concept in our culture is that a man's penis should be like a faucet that can be turned on and off at will. Men and their partners—both straight and gay—assume that the penis can be activated on demand at any time. There will be times and conditions for any man when his organ does not respond. When this does happen, the man may feel incompetent, foolish, and unmanly. His partner might express (verbally or nonverbally) contempt, impatience, and lack of any understanding or sympathy. This can result in trying to force the erection rather than relaxing, breathing, and allowing it to happen. Many partners will be furious when a man masturbates to achieve an erection. They may see this activity as a sign of her or his lack of sexual attraction. Temporary problems with erection can be related to overindulgence in alcohol or drugs, stress at work or home, or exhaustion. There is also performance anxiety, which is especially prevalent if the sexual activity is with a new person. Much of a man's ego depends on: (1) his ability to get an erection on call; (2) the maintenance of that aroused state for a prolonged period of time; and (3) the successful ejaculation.

The opposite problem is an inappropriate erection. It may be because of a relaxed and sensual situation, yet the partner may feel imposed upon and react with anger and/or disgust. I was told a story by one man who had an erection at a nudist colony in the Midwest; he was forced to leave the camp. Spontaneous erections are especially a problem for teenagers and less often as men grow older. Usually they disappear without problem except for the embarrassment. As I have said, when it happens in an older man, the result is an enjoyable feeling no matter where or when it occurs!

There is more public and medical awareness these days of the problem of impotence. This condition is more properly called "erectile dysfunction," a term that is seldom used. The term "impotence" applies to more conditions than the failure of erection of the penis. Previously, it was thought that problems with erection were mostly psychological. As more investigation has occurred, the physical nature of the problem has become more apparent.

Erectile dysfunction may be related to an insufficient arteriole blood supply to the sinuses of the penis. If the sinuses are not distended with sufficient arteriole blood, a partial or no erection will occur. The other major problem occurs when the veins are not blocked off. The blood in the penile sinuses will then be drained too soon. This is often the case when an erection is achieved and cannot be maintained. These conditions can occur as a result of long-term excessive substance abuse or disease. Fortunately, there are current methods to help alleviate the problem (see section 18).

Our culture more or less dictates that a man's arousal must be followed by sexual activity. Women can think that a man's erection means that he will have sex with or without consent. The man assumes that his hard-on must be satisfied by ejaculation. The pleasant feeling of the erect penis itself is ignored. This habit is established in the practice of masturbation when the act is rushed to completion either to avoid detection or to minimize a feeling of guilt. There is no concept of making love to yourself.

I once assumed that married men or men with more or less permanent relationships did not practice masturbation. When I mentioned this to a group of enlightened married men, as a group they rolled their eyes and said "Sure, sure." It was obvious from their expressions that co-habitation does not result in a cessation of masturbation. I hear many men with partners, straight or gay, complain about the frustration of the lack of sex after a period of time. "Spanking the monkey" is an easy, if not as satisfying, answer.

Thus far, I have used the word "ejaculation" rather than "orgasm." The two will generally occur concurrently and yet are two separate responses. Since orgasm and ejaculation generally occur within seconds of one another, it is easy to confuse them. Orgasm includes involuntary rhythmic contraction of the anal sphincter, increased breathing rate, increased heart rate, and elevation of blood pressure. There is a tingling sensation throughout the body. These are changes that occur with a body orgasm. Probably there are many men who experience only a penis orgasm. This occurs when feelings are restricted to the penis and the response of the whole body is nullified by contraction of muscles in general and by holding the breath. Many men have returned to me with big smiles after responding to the suggestion to follow the gymnastics of foreplay with a big breath to relax their body at the time of release. They say that they never knew that an orgasm could be so fulfilling.

Ejaculation has been described as an involuntary muscle spasm, separate from the orgasm—most often indistinguishable. Frequently after ejaculation there is a loss of energy and a feeling of fatigue. It is taken for granted that ejaculation drains a man's energy. Athletes have been known to abstain from ejaculating before a contest. It is a cultural joke about the man who ejaculates, grunts, and collapses, leaving his partner unsatisfied. Sometimes this is preceded by a rush to the bathroom to wash off the "dirty" semen. This is a demonstration of the negative attitude toward a natural secretion of the body. When the genital/anal region is regarded with guilt or distaste, anything coming from it is immediately washed off. I have often thought that men should wash their hands before uri-nating rather than after. The penis has fewer germs than the outside world.

Premature ejaculation is often related to performance anxiety or a rapid response to a sensuous touch. I once worked with a man who told me that when he first came to see me he hated being touched by a man. When I asked him why he was here, he said it was because his wife and therapist (both of whom I had Rolfed) talked him into it. When we came to the session that focused on the abdomen, he became erect and ejacu-lated as soon as I touched the area. He was very embarrassed, and I trust that I hid my surprise. I assured him that this had happened before (it was the first but not the last time). The following session these events hap-pened when I touched a little lower on his abdomen. He asked me why I had to work on such an erotic area. I told him that the entire body could be erotic. In later sessions, I was able to work on his pubic bone with a resultant erection and no ejaculation. Finally I could work around the genital region with no response. My impression was that the man suf-fered from premature ejaculation because his body had not had much touching. Therefore any touching was erotic to him. When we finished I asked him how he felt about the work. His response was, "I don't hate being touched by a man anymore." I later found out that he quit his ther-apist and his wife got pregnant.

It is possible for men to have orgasms without ejaculation. This is part of the Taoist, Tantric, and Sufi traditions. Sexual Kung Fu was developed in Chinese medicine as a health benefit by the Taoist masters. This basi-cally is non-ejaculatory orgasm—something not considered in our cul-ture. Some men can have multiple ejaculations during one love-making session (especially teenage boys), which is quite different from multiple non-ejaculatory orgasms. The erotic release of the tingling, almost elec-tric, sensation of the orgasm need not be followed by the pumping action of ejaculation. A man can be trained to enjoy the orgasm in and of itself. Without the exhaustion effects of ejaculation, orgasms can be repeated.

The concept of multiple orgasms, orgasm without ejaculation, leads to the possibility of repetition of orgasms. Our concept of "getting horny" is what the Taoists thought of as generating sexual energy for life. The sex-ual or erotic energy goes upwards into the body and is used as functional energy, rather than being expelled as semen. This involves understanding the various erotic areas of the body. The penis is obvious, as are the testicles, although sometimes the erogenous aspect of the testicles is not appreciated. There are men whose testicles are so painful to the touch to a point that stroking them will be a turn-off.

The perineum is an area considered "dirty" or disgusting by many men. There was a period when I took Polaroid® pictures of men's perineum to educate them on the part of their anatomy they couldn't see. A negative response was quite usual. I discontinued the practice when I discovered that my intention was sometimes misinterpreted. This is an area which contains the base of the penis; the prostate lies immediately underneath. This can be one of the erotic areas when the mind set is open. When the penis is habitually drawn in by protective responses, much of the base of the penis may be felt by palpation in the perineum.

The prostate can be erotic at the time of arousal. There is often a negative attitude about this gland because of the pain and discomfort of rectal examinations. This ties in with other negative attitudes about the anus.

The pubococcygeus or PC muscle (a part of the levator ani complex) is a muscular sling connecting the coccyx to the back of the pubic bone at the base of the penis. It is said to be responsible for the rhythmic contractions of the pelvis and anus during orgasm. It surrounds the prostate and serves as a valve around the genitals. It is also a factor in urine control. With lack of use, the muscle may lose its tone, which will decrease sexual function and pleasure. There are exercises to reestablish the function of the muscle. These exercises, called the Kegel exercises, have been applied to women. It seems logical that they would be of benefit to men's sexual activity also. To my knowledge this has not been investigated.

The anus with its high concentration of sensitive nerve endings is also a highly erogenous zone. Many people consider it "unnatural" to stimulate the anus. I have had several straight men come to me upset after finding that they enjoyed having their anus touched. I have assured them that this in no way meant that they were gay. Since there is a direct connection of the external anal sphincter to the perineum and thus to the "genital muscles," frequent contraction of the anus is an inhibitory factor in the enjoyment of normal sexual function by pulling in the base of the penis.

The nipples are another erogenous zone in many men. There can be negative feelings about this as being feminine. The body as a whole can be erogenous—a back rub can cause arousal. Most men are too blocked about their bodies to allow these feelings. There is the problem of any touching being considered sexual.

Recently there has been rather startling information on the relation between cycling and impotency.* Dr. Irwin Goldstein of Boston University Medical Center estimates that there are about 100,000 men who have lost the ability to get or to maintain satisfactory erections because of penile damage inflicted by either the narrowness of the bike's seat or the bar in men's bikes. Prolonged time spent on a bicycle can result in injury and scarring of the arteries which provide the blood for erections. The narrow seat of men's bicycles presses on the perineum, which contains about 50% of the penis. At times, the entire body weight rests on this area. This is true also for stationary bikes where the man tends to sit and peddle. This concept has not been met with enthusiasm in these days of bicycling being promoted as one of the best forms of cardiovascular exercise. Dr. Goldstein's suggestion is that the seats for men be made wider with more padding.

I mentioned this to a friend of mine in his fifties who was having problems with erections. I knew that he cycled several miles each day for exercise. He recently told me that after giving up riding the bicycle for several weeks, his erections were much better and the numbness between his legs had disappeared. His concern was how to exercise without hurting himself. The purchase of a special wider seat with a depressed midsection seems to have solved the problem.

---

*Kita, Joe, "Impotency and Cycling: The Unseen Danger." *Bicycling,* Aug. 1997.

10

Touching

MANY YEARS AGO I attended a lecture given by a rather militant female therapist. She was addressing her comments to male Rolfers about their lack of sensitivity to their female clients. She stated that most women had not been touched by a man except for sex. I thought that she was blatantly overstating her case. I mentioned this to my female clients. Without exception they agreed with her. Each of them said that the Rolfing sessions were the first time that they had been touched by a man except for sex!

Most of my male clients, both straight and gay, complain that they seldom get touched, especially in the pelvic region. This seems to be true even in long-term relationships where touching in general becomes less and less frequent with time. In many cases, sex becomes a ritual rather than a pleasure.

The amount of touching in general is related to the culture. The Latin and Mediterranean cultures have much more touching between men. They may hug, kiss, and walk down the street with arms around each other. I have seen Russian men walk hand in hand. Male to male touching is completely foreign to the northern European cultures. The French kiss-kiss on the cheeks is done as though from a distance. The touching of pelvis to pelvis, which I have heard called "gourmet hugging," is considered too threatening or suggestive.

Touch is the first sense developed in the embryo. It is said to be present at about the beginning of the second month of pregnancy. The other sense organs develop much later. The skin is exposed to the soothing feel of the amniotic fluid surrounding the developing embryo and fetus. This pleasant sensation is abruptly terminated at time of birth.

There have been efforts to modify the harshness of the treatment of the baby after the birth. Some methods place the baby in water to simulate the amniotic fluid. This is not generally used today due to the possibility of contamination of the water. It is more common for the naked babies to be placed next to the skin of the mother to begin bonding. The materials used to wrap the baby come from the hospital laundry and have the corresponding rough texture. In home birth, softer materials no doubt are used. New skin thermometers are replacing the insult to the anus by rectal thermometers. There have been more attempts to humanize post-birth procedures. It will vary from region to region and hospital to hospital.

The attitudes that develop during childhood will to a large part depend on the nonverbal messages from the family and surrounding culture. Part of the character development will involve one's attitude about touch. A correlation is the fact that when young, children will look directly into a person's eyes. Most adults cannot handle this and will avert their eyes. The child learns without any verbal message that direct eye contact is not desirable and withdraws. Likewise, they will learn to desist from touching or being touched. This is especially true for boys; touching in girls is considered more appropriate.

This is a generational condition which in turn has been a response to culture. In many parts of this country, families are very close emotionally and yet touching is limited to a handshake or a pat on the back. Any more demonstrative touching will result in a flinch, a holding of the breath, and a subtle physical withdrawal by deadening the area. Physical withdrawal will be accompanied by emotional withdrawal. These will be strong factors in character development.

I have mentioned how many parents are inhibited about touching the genitals. As soon as the boy is old enough, he is handed a washcloth and told to wash himself "down there." The Catholic doctrine I have heard is that he must always use a cloth—never his bare hand. This lack of touch-

ing of the genitalia and anus continues throughout childhood. The pleasure of the area by touch is not developed. This is a fine line since boys
usually have sexual fantasies about their mother, their father, or both. The
fear would be that these fantasies might be enhanced and thus cause misunderstanding. These days the fear of accusations of sexual abuse must
make parents even more careful about touching in the pelvic region.

There is the stage where a young boy becomes modest, usually about
his genitals and less frequently about his anal region. One man told me
about being washed in a basin of water warmed by a wood stove when
he was very young. He was more modest about his rear while his mother
kept insisting that he turn his front away from the watching public of
grandmother and aunts. He was toilet trained very young. His negative
attitude about shit and the anus, as demonstrated by wanting to keep his
buttocks covered, was already established.

These areas become "touchy." Nonsexual touching almost anywhere
on the buttocks and especially near the tailbone will result in an automatic squeezing of the gluteals together. This can also happen during sex.
The response is often not conscious. In the front, the groin and pubic areas
are particularly susceptible to "don't touch me." The sensation may be a
tickle, a feeling of anger, or the comment that "It just feels funny." Some
men are sensitive in their entire abdominal region. Neutral touch anywhere in the area will result in a flinching which is a tightening plus a
holding of the breath. Both the tightening and breath-holding are methods to repress sensation. One Rolfer told me that his father absolutely
refused to let him touch his abdomen during the Rolfing. No amount of
coercion worked. What can one say to one's father?

These protective patterns exist in both gay and straight men. The
assumption is that they develop pre-sexually, if such a condition exists.
A woman Rolfer who worked exclusively on children told me that children are indeed sexual beings from an early age.

Teenage boys are likely to resist touch. As the hormonal effects become
more pronounced and confusing, the light touch of a mother or female
relative can cause embarrassing feelings and the fear of a penis response.
By this time fathers also avoid touching their sons altogether except for
an occasional pat on the back or the butt. This could begin to establish a

pattern of not touching females except for sex and touching other males in only a rough fashion.

There exists the idea that young people were more free with touch and sex in the 1960s and 1970s. This was proclaimed the "sexual revolution." Back in the early 1970s, I spent a week at the Esalen Institute on the California coast. I left there full of the ecstasy from a week of freedom to touch and a liberation of the feelings in my body. I picked up a young hitchhiker and was extolling how wonderful it must be to grow up at that period of time. His jolting comment was: "We may have more sex but our relationships are not any better!"

My impression today is that many of those young people who were so free back then have reverted to a more conservative attitude with time and the need to provide for their living. The young men that I work on now, the sons of men of that era, are more modest about their bodies and more hesitant about touch than older men. Has there been a reversal to bring children up in the same manner that was revolted against in the past? Has the pendulum swung back?

It is certainly simplistic to relate this to breathing. Yet, many of the spiritual leaders of that time were influenced by Eastern practices which involved focusing on the breath. When faced with the reality and stress of practical living, breathing takes a second place. The usual response to thinking and doing is holding the breath. This affects the flow of body movement.

The holding of the breath effectively cuts off sensations not only into the pelvis but in the whole body. The breath-holding can also be localized. Certain areas can be "cut off" whether due to pain or to the fear of pleasure. The tickle is "don't touch me here." The tickle response is to squirm and hold the breath—like jumping into cold water. It is my impression that ticklishness hides erotic areas. One man reported that all of his life he had been extremely ticklish under his armpits and on the bottoms of his feet. During Rolfing he was encouraged not to hold his breath when these areas were being touched. Eventually he found these to be among the most pleasurable and sensual areas of his body.

Permission to touch changes in a sexual situation. Sometimes it seems as though a switch has been turned on—or perhaps the lights are turned off. It is suddenly O.K. to hug, to kiss, to fondle, to stroke any place in the body. It's like a conditioned response, perhaps like Pavlov's dog, who started to salivate when food was presented.

Sexual touching, however, can be very limited. With gay men it is not unusual for there to be a single focus—the penis. This remains true whether one wants his penis attended to by the other or is the one focused on pleasing his partner. At least one penis must be erect and ready to function. In some cases, the partner will not make any effort to stimulate arousal. They seem to feel that their very presence should serve as sufficient stimulus.

A short interaction with the nipples may be tried since some men are extremely sensitive and may respond with an erection by that method. The anus may be touched, particularly if anal penetration is the goal. It is a focus on sex, not love-making. The problem here is a combination of the two backgrounds with the cultural inhibitions about men touching or being touched. There is also the guilt coming from negative family and cultural attitudes about homosexuality. The feelings in many gay men consist of rebellion mixed with shame.

One may assume that straight couples are more liberated these days. The message I get is that the discussions about sex are more open, yet the touching is not much changed. A number of young men with relationships have mentioned that they seldom get touched in the pelvic region. One man related that he had been married for fifteen years. During that time, it was his responsibility to motivate his wife for sex. This took much time and alcohol. By the time she was ready, he was no longer interested or able, which made her very angry. Never once in fifteen years did his wife initiate sex or touch his penis.

Wives and female companions complain about the lack of sensitivity of their male mates. The main issue is the man's focus on penetration and ejaculation. Often little attempt is made to satisfy the woman physically or emotionally. Since men are trained with strong nonverbal messages that sensuality is not appropriate for a man, it is easy to understand why he is not aware of that need in his female companion. Love-making is not in his repertoire. He has dulled physical sensation in all of his body except the penis. My image is a metal diaper with an opening for the penis. The result is that his orgasms are localized and often unsatisfactory. The man can blame his partner and look for more fulfillment elsewhere, not realizing that the problem is his, not his partner's. This can also be true for the "top" in a gay relationship.

The basis of these protections and inhibitions is the fear of intimacy. Touching involves responsibility. Some people can touch and not be available to receive touch. Others enjoy being touched and cannot bring themselves to reciprocate. Sensual touching (as opposed to sexual) indicates an intimacy. The intimacy in turn can cause a feeling of vulnerability and the fear of loss of autonomy or independence. There is also the fear of misinterpretation. It is safer not to demonstrate sensitivity in this way.

I read once that a woman's idea of a relationship is face to face; a man's idea is side by side. A best-selling book some years ago concerned secrets that men keep. The secret was that men have feelings!

11

Pelvic Movement

AN OLDER WOMAN who freely admits to many sexual liaisons in her past told me that of all the men she had been with, only one had been satisfying sexually. He was not the best-looking man nor did he have the best body. She felt that when they were having sex, he had a rhythm to the movement of his pelvis. The other men, including two ex-husbands, had been very stiff in their pelvic movement.

The pelvic movement in men, or lack thereof, can be readily observed in porno movies. In the missionary position, most men are doing "push-ups" with little or no movement between the pelvis and the lower back. The entire body is moving up and down. When the man is on his back there will be a lifting of the entire lower body if there is any movement at all. There is very little sensation in the pelvis except for the penis.

Occasionally there will be the contrast of a man moving his pelvis in a thrusting motion. The hips will rock forward led by the pubic bone. There will be flexibility in the lower back. When these men are on their back, there will be a rocking motion in the pelvis where the tailbone slides down while the pubic bone moves headward. The lower back lengthens and the abdominal muscles contract. In these cases the pelvis is free and feelings can reverberate throughout the body before as well as during the orgasm.

The pattern of rigidity in the lower back and pelvis could have been established by frantic and hurried masturbation in the early years. Often those regions were held rigid to speed up the process to the desired orgasm and ejaculation. This will usually be accompanied by holding the breath, especially at the time of orgasm, localizing the sensation.

Publicly, the best way to observe pelvic movement is to watch a man dance. There is an assumption that Caucasian men do not get the beat of the music while Black men and Latinos do. This generalization has not been my observation. There are, of course, variations from culture to culture—mostly individual differences in movement.

In any dance step, the pelvic movement is essential to respond to the rhythm. Often men look like robots jumping up and down. The pelvis does not move in isolation. It is sometimes helpful to look at the body with the idea of suspension. The shoulders are suspended from the neck, and the arms from the shoulders. These are the easiest parts of the body to envision with this model. It is also possible to consider the pelvis suspended from the chest and abdomen, and the legs being suspended from the pelvis. The body can be envisioned as a puppet on strings. When one part is moved, the entire body responds. If a part is held rigid, the entire movement is affected.

In dance, it is not that the pelvis must move on its own but rather that it is moved in rhythm with the rest of the body. In flamenco dance, I am told by a dance teacher, the movement originates in the lower chest with smooth movement progressing through the pelvis to the legs like a type of swaying suspension. The pelvic action and reaction is a basic part of the beauty of Latin American dance (samba, rumba, salsa, reggae) and African dance. Even jitterbug and disco are more pleasing with the pelvis engaged. In jitterbug dancing, the man is often walking around, spinning his partner here and there. Many men dancing to disco music are mainly jumping up and down with great enthusiasm and abandon but little rhythm.

Many years ago after my first series of Rolfing, I was invited to a church dance on Sunday afternoon. The band was a trio of old-timers playing rocking jitterbug music. After the first dance, my partner refused to dance with me again because the way I was moving my hips was "immoral." I was upset because it felt so freeing.

Considering what we might call performance dance, ballet and modern, the pelvis is stationary. It is not to be moved when the top of the body or the legs are in motion. The hips are "square." When the pelvis is moved, it is moved as a block. A variation is African dance, where the hips are moved freely.

Smooth movement of the pelvis does not mean bump and grind. There are some occasions where this could be appropriate. Very few men can activate the pelvis sufficiently to do that motion. This entails not only loosening up the structure of the lower back and abdomen but also freeing up inhibitions.

I have heard slow dancing referred to as sex standing up. I was told of an old Mennonite joke that the reason the Mennonites do not have sex standing is that it might lead to dancing. This is an example of how any touching or sensual movement of the pelvis has to have a sexual connotation. It rules out the possibility that men can just be sexual/sensual *per se* rather than always thinking that the sex act must be the goal.

Pelvic restriction affects many other movements of the body: walking, running, jumping, sports, aerobics, etc. The pelvis can be thought of as similar to a baby's cradle. The pelvis is suspended by the heads of the femurs. It has the possibility of rocking like a cradle. The rocking is subtle and from front to back—not side to side. This movement is often inhibited in the back by the clenching of the buttocks (tight ass) and/or the tightening and shortening of the lower back, the lumbar region. There also may be a grabbing or pulling up in the groin area in front. These will lock the pelvis in an immobile state. The restrictions can be alleviated by focused breathing down to the perineum and permission to "let go." Sometimes it is necessary to focus either to the back or front, depending on the area protected.

Other areas of the body will likewise affect the movement of the pelvis. The contracted abdomen, often reinforced by many sit-ups, will pull down the chest and shorten the distance between the chest and the pubic bone. Most people have worries about their protruding abdomen and hold on to it for dear life. It seems to be a factor in personal, business, and social behavior. A rigid abdomen is an indication of a rigid person.

Shoulder movement affects the movement of the pelvis. One can tell the difference in walking. If the arms and shoulders are allowed to swing freely, the pelvis moves. If the shoulders are held quiet by putting your hands in your pockets, the movement of the pelvis is much more restricted. People with lower back pain will find it exacerbated by carrying something heavy where the arm and shoulder movements are restricted.

The swinging motion of alternate arms and legs allows for a cross-pattern of movement between the shoulders and the pelvis. Thus the right shoulder will move forward with the left side of the pelvis and vice versa. The two sides of the pelvis are held together by supposedly "slightly" movable joints. Actually those joints can allow for a subtle back-and-forth movement of the two sides.

Everyone has a body rotation where the shoulders and chest face in one direction and the pelvis faces the other. In walking or running, the leg on the side of the pelvis that is more forward has the least distance to go. The leg on the side of the pelvis that is back has to swing around from behind. This will result in a slightly uneven gait characteristic to each person.

Most of us hold our head and neck still when we are thinking or performing some action. This means that when walking the vibration set up by the feet hitting the ground will be stopped at the neck, causing headaches among other symptoms. If one walks with the head rocking in response to the movement and then holds the head very still while continuing to walk, one can feel the inhibition of movement throughout the entire body. The head movement is a response, not an active function like the rocking motion of the pelvis.

The first step in opening up movement of the pelvis is to give oneself permission to feel that area, with the endpoint being just awareness. The effect can come from within by breathing into the area and from without as response to gentle touch. This is actually one of the methods used in the treatment of impotence. The principle is to have the sensation without performance anxiety. The prevailing attitude is that it is improper to feel in that area except when having sex. Some might consider this awareness to be immoral.

The next step is to take that feeling into movement. Feel where you tighten once the movement is initiated. If there is an area of chronic pain, that area usually will tighten more in movement. For example, people with lower back problems may be able to allow for movement in that area in walking. Once they start to run, however, there often is a protective tightening in the lower back, pulling up the buttocks. This in turn cuts off any possibility of pelvic movement as well as increases the degree of pain. Unfortunately, this is the usual body response to pain. We tighten the area, creating more pain, and stop our breath on the inhale. The recommended response is to complete the breath with a good exhale—something easier said than done.

Another factor, especially in running in men, is protection of the genitals. There appears to be the fear of damage when they are "hanging loose." Jock straps, dance belts, or tight undershorts worn over a long period of time can cause irritation to both the penis and the scrotum, to say nothing of what these garments do to the sperm count.

The big problem is our cultural lack of the concept to "allow" anything to occur. We are a "doing" society. Anything that is worthwhile must be worked at. The usual response I get from a male client when I suggest that he feel an area or movement in that area is "I'll work at it." To relax and feel something is beyond their comprehension. This is the first teaching, the first permission.

12

Protection

O NE ASPECT OF PROTECTION is modesty—always covering the genitals. This may start during the juvenile years as a reaction to family and/or peers. There will be the effect of the parents' modesty. Some families come to breakfast fully dressed at all times. There will never be exposure to the rest of the family in nightclothes or robes. The movement in and out of the bathroom will be done surreptitiously. Instructions might be given to put toilet paper in the bowl before urinating to lessen the sound or to run the water in the sink. How many boys have peed outside the toilet in the effort to hit the area of the bowl around the edge of the water? The natural noises of elimination are to be muffled.

Gas emitted during bowel movements can cause embarrassment if the bathroom walls are thin. Often the anus will be squeezed to "sneak out" the farts. This does not facilitate easy bowel movements.

Years ago there were group showers in gymnasiums. Boys and men swam in the nude in YMCA pools and school pools. Often the only clothing requirement was a bathing cap for those with longer hair. Dressing rooms were open without curtains. Sometimes the toilet stalls did not have doors or, in the Army, no stalls at all. In the armed forces, men slept on cots close together, sometimes naked in hot weather before air conditioning. Draft physicals were a very leveling experience. Men walked around in briefs, lowering them before everyone to have their genital area checked for hernias and then leaning over and spreading their cheeks to be checked for hemorrhoids. It was impossible to be modest in front of other men under these crude circumstances.

Things have changed over the years. Bathing suits are now required in most pools, even in an all male environment. Health clubs have individual dressing rooms. The showers are cubicles with curtains. Draft physicals, thank goodness, are a thing of the past. I have noticed that younger men seem to be much more uncomfortable nude in front of other men (dancers excepted) than their elders. It may be more unusual for them to be so.

The protective gesture of the hands over the genitals is not uncommon. While standing, the hands are clasped together in front of the genitals (Fig. 12-1). This is especially true when men are nude. Even more common is this gesture when sitting in public places. I notice on the subways of NYC, 90% of the men have their hands or coats draped over their genitals, a newspaper or bag sitting on their lap, or they are leaning forward on their elbows so that the genitals are pushed back and covered (Fig. 12-2).

Many men will make great effort to hide their penis in public. At urinals, they will stand in a broad stance and thrust their hips forward so that the penis is hidden inside the urinal. There is covering with the hands by forming a tube with the fingers around the penis. There is an internal pushing to force the urine out. The contrast which is occasionally seen is a man standing very relaxed allowing the urine to flow.

In locker rooms, some men will change their clothes with the front of their body hidden behind the door of the locker. They may find a place next to a wall and do all of their rapid changing with their back to the room. Towels can be used as a curtain to cover. In public baths, there will be men who cover themselves with towels or shorts. Often during bodywork on a table, some men seem comfortable being naked. As soon as they get up, however, the protective gesture to cover the genitals with their hands will occur and they will grab for their shorts (Fig. 12-1).

Some modesty comes from family and cultural background. Another

FIGURE 12-1 ➤

Protective gestures when naked

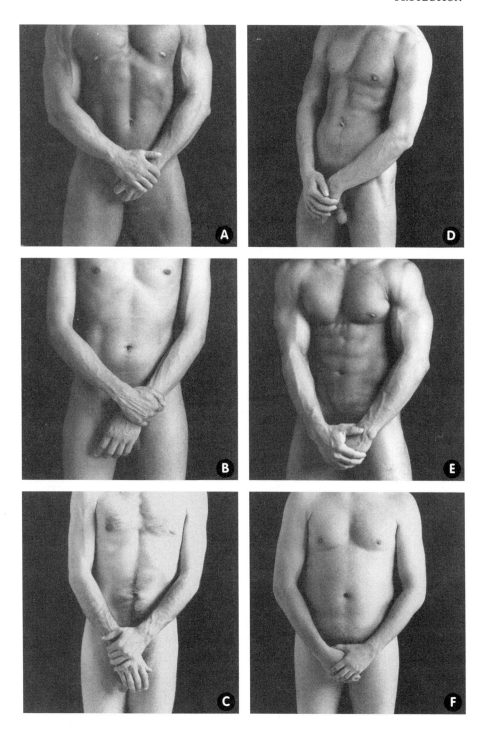

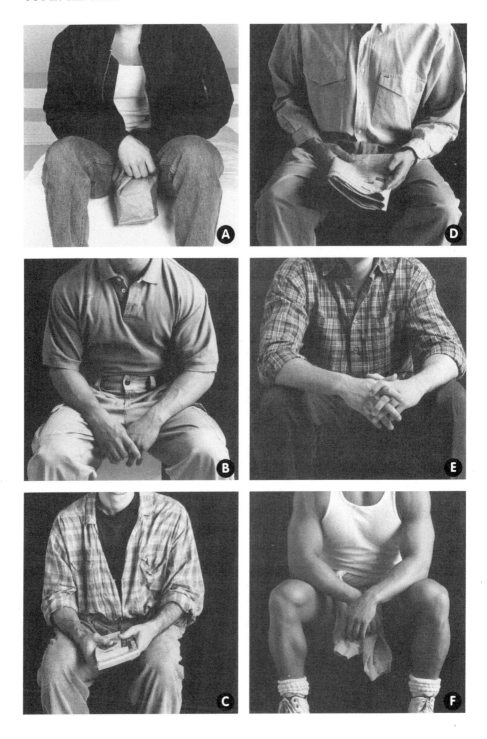

factor is the wish not to have any comparison on size or shape. I have seldom found a man who did not wish that his penis was bigger. There is the possible fear of an embarrassing erection. I know one man whose wife felt that she owned his penis. He was forbidden to have anyone else see it. He never changed his clothes in public. In public restrooms, he used the cubicles.

The type of clothing a man chooses demonstrates his opinion about his body. Some men will wear loose to baggy attire to obscure their body in such a way that no one has any idea what it looks like. This seems especially true of boys today. Other men wear such tight garments that there is no question of their manhood and muscular development. It may be selective—tight top and loose bottom or the reverse. A man told me that on nude beaches in California, he was not at all modest about his genitals. He was very aware of his protruding belly and thus he wore loose tops with no bottom on the beach.

There is the internal method of protection, which has already been discussed to some extent. The muscles at the base of the penis may pull the organ in with habitual contraction. There can be one to three inches of the penis pulled inside the perineum. The habitual contraction of those muscles can also cause a man to become "pee shy." It is not possible for him to relax the muscles to allow the urine to flow in public.

One of the ways to strengthen the pubococcygeus muscle is to consciously interrupt the urine flow by intermittent contraction and relaxation. It would seem that men who have problems urinating in public cannot relax the muscle under those conditions. When they try, they hold their breath on the inhale in their effort to push out the urine rather than relaxing with the exhale, which allows for easier flow.

There is a series of horizontal fascial bands or straps across the body. One of the most prominent lies across the inguinal region or the groin. It is like a jock strap under the skin. When overly tight, it will restrict the breath from reaching the area below. This restriction will numb the feeling of that area. This band is especially apparent in men with large bellies

---

◄ FIGURE 12-2

Common protective postures in public

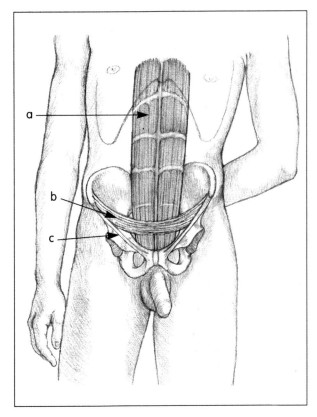

FIGURE 12-3
Pelvic band
(a) rectus abdominus (b) pelvic band
(c) inguinal ligament

and very slender hips. It's as though the band forms a support for the oversized abdomen. These men constantly have to "hitch up their pants." This structure, which is a modification of the fascial bed, can also be seen in small children. It will become reinforced over the years by the habitual lack of breathing and the internal restriction for protection. The band will be where most men wear their pants. It is like a comfort zone (Figs. 12-3, 12-4).

While men can be very preoccupied with their penis, many of them feel almost apologetic about their butts. On nude beaches I notice that women walk around as though proud of their derrieres. Men, on the other hand, walk as though they were ashamed of that part of their body. It gives the appearance of covering it without physically doing so.

The traditional Charles Atlas concept of the perfect male body still exists. The goal is large chest and shoulders, small hips, and large thighs. When these relative proportions are in excess, the pelvis cannot properly function as a conduit between the large masses above and below. It can be compared to a tube of toothpaste being squeezed in the middle,

FIGURE 12-4 ➤
Front views
Note the variations in the pelvic bands.

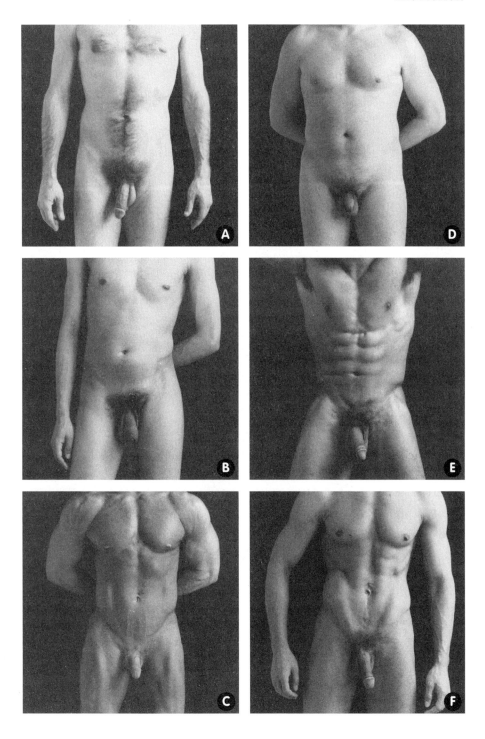

the top and bottom bulging out. The only recourse for a bodyworker is to try to stabilize and keep the balance of the body. These proportions often inhibit graceful or sensual movement through the pelvis.

There can be the conscious or unconscious concept that squeezing the buttocks will make the hips smaller. This not only cuts off feeling and movement, it pushes the tissue headward and may be a factor in the problem of excessive "love handles." If we think of tissue being able to flow like lava, relaxing the buns will allow the tissue to flow from the hips down into the thighs and thus more effectively reduce the size of the hips.

This tightness of the buttocks is even more apparent when a man leans over. The gluteals remain tightly clamped rather than the tuberosities or sitz bones widening. Accompanying this is the increased contraction of the anal sphincters. This reaction can be due to the fear of being unclean or of committing the social error of passing gas. The tightening is especially true if the man is nude (Fig. 12-5).

When doing bodywork, there are times when it can be appropriate for a man to raise both legs while lying on his back. This position facilitates work on the hamstring muscles, the lower gluteus maximus, and the perineum. Many times this will provoke feelings of discomfort and vulnerability. A number of men have commented: "I have not been in this position since I was a baby." There will be a varying degree of "covering the anus" by squeezing the hamstrings and the gluteus maximus (Fig. 12-6).

I have noticed while doing bodywork that trust must be established before working on the protected areas of the body. After this has been accomplished, it is not unusual for a man to drift off into "twilight zone" and for his penis to become aroused when the pubic area is worked on. Likewise, the same state can be reached when the buttocks are being worked on and they will relax. These responses will frequently be reversed when the habitual state of consciousness is regained.

The cutting off of feeling to the pelvis can be quite complete. The genital area may become so insensitive that the penis can be erect without

FIGURE 12-5 ➤

Varying degrees of "tight ass"
The figures are arranged from the most protected anus (A) to the most open (F).

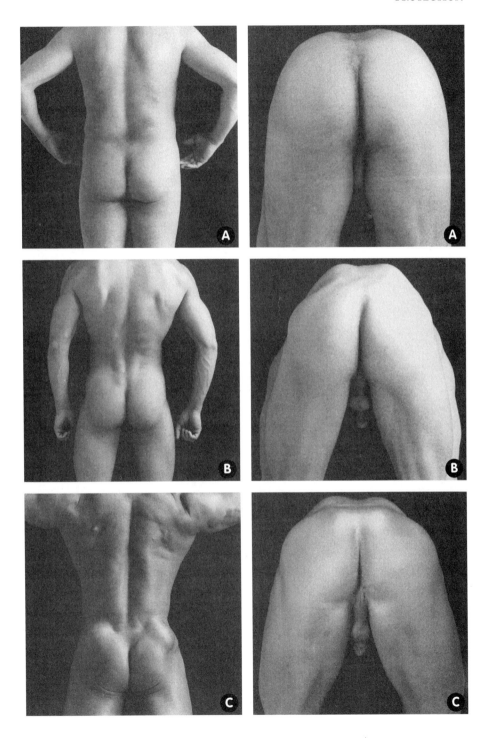

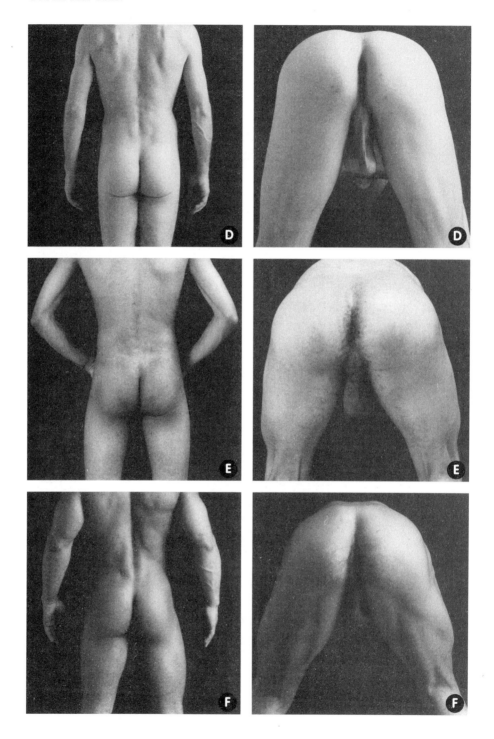

the person being aware. I have seen men's testicles squeezed between their thighs with no apparent discomfort. The perineum can become like concrete with no response to gentle touching. The buttocks are frequently squeezed tight and rub together to the point that there is irritation between the cheeks with no awareness.

The summary of protection is "Don't move it, don't feel it, don't breathe into it, cover it." It doesn't exist if you pretend it's not there!

◄ FIGURE 12-5 (CONT.)

Note that the degree of anal protection is relatively independent of the tightness of the muscles of the back.

FIGURE 12-6 ➤

Openness of the perineal/anal region with the legs raised
The figures are arranged from the most protected (A) to the most open (F).

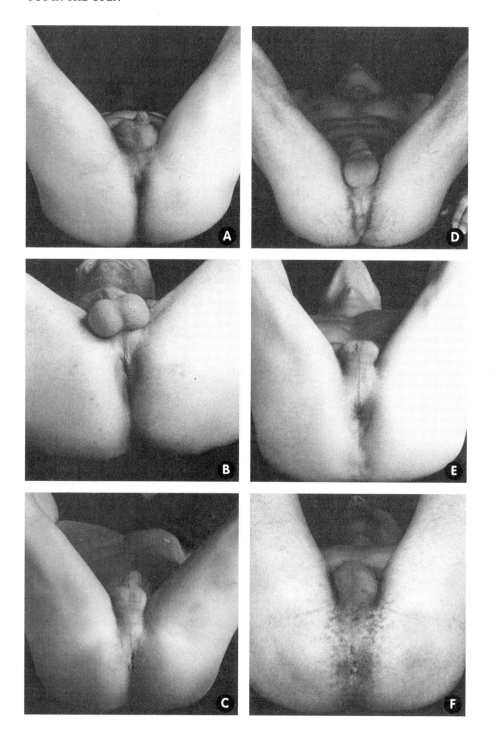

13

Habit Patterns

I N DOING AN EVALUATION of protective structural patterns in men, it is necessary to keep in mind that everyone is an individual. What is being pointed out are general impressions obtained from years of observations and touching, as a professional Rolfer. The degree of restrictions will vary from man to man.

The unique factor in men is the presence of external genitalia and the resulting self-defense. Often men seem to have the entire trunk of the body pulled down in front. This differs from women's bodies, which seem to just sag internally rather than an active pulling down (information I have received from women Rolfers). The impression is that the penis acts like a hook. When it is pulled in, it serves to pull the front or center (core) of the body down. When the clenching of the penis is relieved by a combination of awareness, permission, and breathing and the penis hangs free, the body can then "spring" up (Fig. 13-1).

The defense in movement is to walk "around" the genitals. The legs will move in walking while the pubic region remains static. There is no consciousness of the genitals in walking or running and certainly no breath going down to that region. It is always

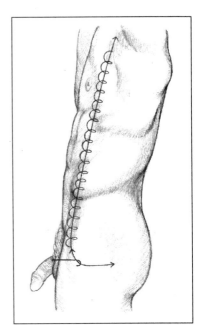

FIGURE 13-1
Penis "hook" and body spring

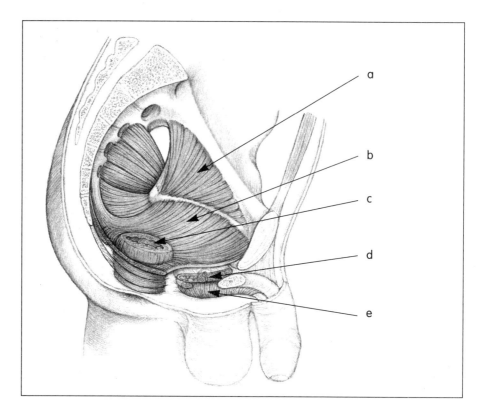

FIGURE 13-2
Pelvic muscles
(a) iliacus m. (b) levator ani m. (c) anal canal (d) perineal m.
(e) muscles of the penis

a surprise to my client when I touch the rami between the legs and tell them that this is the bottom of their abdomen. There are two diaphragms (the pelvic and the urogenital) in that area which serve in concert as the base of the abdominal breathing (Fig. 13-2). When this area is liberated to feeling, the genitals can move with the rest of the body.

The movement should be through the center of the pelvis rather than around it. I suggest that the man feel the bouncing of the genitalia when he walks. This, of course is more difficult with tight briefs or jeans. An exercise I suggest is to feel the genitals bounce when walking around naked. A man can check the movement of the genitals by looking in a mirror if he cannot feel it.

In many men, there is a pulling in of the inner thighs—sometimes to the point where they rub together. In the extreme, it creates a persistent irritation and the reddish appearance of a rash. This habit could have come from the persistent use of the inner thighs as an adjunct to the bladder muscles. It is not only a pulling in but also a drawing up of those adductor muscles. The fascia of the adductor muscles (inner thigh) will be continuous with that of the perineum (urogenital diaphragm) and thus with the fascia of the muscles at the base of the penis. This supplements the habitual contraction of the penile musculature (Fig. 13-3).

Habitual contraction of the muscles of the inner thigh will naturally cause a response on the rest of the leg as well as the rest of the body. The pulling on the inner thigh will result in tension on the outside of the thigh. There will be a compensatory action of the gluteus maximus and the tensor fascia lata, whose extension is the iliotibial tract which lines the outside of the thigh (see Fig. 8-1). This will shorten the distance between the

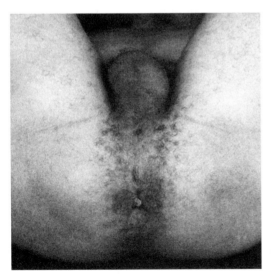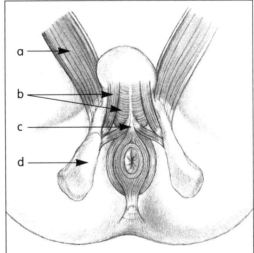

FIGURE 13-3

Continuity of adductor muscles with urogenital diaphragm (perineum)
(a) gracilis m. (adductor m.) (b) muscles of the penis (c) transverse perineal m.
(d) ramus

pelvis and the knee, possibly causing the lower leg to splay out from the knee.

The hamstrings will respond by shortening and pulling up, which in turn pulls down the lower border of the gluteus maximus. Although the hamstrings are not directly adjacent to the maximus, their fascia is continuous with the underside of the lower border. The fascia of the hamstrings is also continuous with that of the perineum and can act to narrow the space between the tuberosities.

The quadriceps muscles on the front of the leg may then be pulled up into the groin region. The overall effect is that of pulling the entire leg up into the pelvis and shortening it. These compensations inhibit the free movement of the femur in the socket of the pelvis (acetabulum) and create a stiff walk. The stiffness of walking creates pressure above the groin, increasing the density of the band crossing that area (see Fig. 12-3). This band and the resultant lack of movement cut off the possibility and probability of breathing and feeling in there. The feelings that may become apparent include pain from strain in the area where the adductor muscles meet the rami (beside the testicles), the inguinal region, and/or the hip joints.

In the back there is the protection of the buttocks and anus, which also involves the lower back. At the more external level, the gluteus maximus can be held so tight that the cheeks rub against each other. The anal sphincters will also be habitually contracted in this situation, even during bowel movements. The entire cleft between the buttocks looks inflamed. The area will be sweaty. These cheeks do not spread when the man leans over or sits down (Fig. 12-5). It seems probable that these men would suffer from constipation. A number of men have commented to me that after they have more feeling of openness in the buttocks, they no longer need a library in the bathroom. The strain in bowel movements is lessened if not relieved entirely.

At a deeper level in the buttocks, the lateral rotators are often very tight and can feel like cables under the maximus. This will create the dimple or depression on the sides of the buttocks. Since these muscles converge on the back of the greater trochanter of the femur, their tightening can create a backward pull on the bone, causing it to rotate in the joint.

This results in a fairly common "duck walk" (especially favored by ballet dancers).

My initial impression was that if the buttocks were tucked under, the genitals would be thrust forward. Conversely, if the genitals were hanging low between the legs, the butt would stick out in back. These relationships can be seen in many men. There are cases, however, where both the butt and genitals are tucked under. It is as though the anus and penis are drawn together by the tissue being pulled up between the rami into the body (Fig. 13-4). My image is a napkin being pulled through a napkin ring. Examining the anatomy of the area demonstrates that this can happen. The two diaphragms would be a major factor. Both have intimate muscular and fascial attachments to the base of the penis and the anal sphincters. Habitual tightening of the perineum (urogenital diaphragm) and the levator ani (pelvic diaphragm) will pull the anus and the penis closer together and literally up into the body. The variation in the degree of contraction also explains the differences in the distance between the anus and the base of the penis in different men.

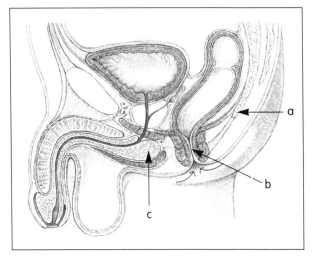

FIGURE 13-4
Saggital section of the male pelvis
(a) coccyx (b) anal canal (c) base of the penis
(arrows indicate direction of tissue pull in tight ass).

14

Body Work

THIS SECTION IS FOR BODYWORKERS to give them an idea of how to approach the work around the male genitals, if it is indicated. *This work should be done only if the bodyworker is comfortable with his/her own sexuality and is comfortable with the client!*

Restrictive habit patterns can be modified by a combination of sensitive movement techniques and equally sensitive body work. Both involve working with the breath (see Appendix II). The first step is to "wake up" the region, to increase awareness. Since both the anal region and the groin are "don't touch me" areas, trust of the man for both himself and for the therapist must be well established.

In working with the pelvis, one must constantly remember that the area does not exist in isolation. There are muscle connections to the legs and trunk as well as fascial and muscle relationships to the entire body. Tightness in the shoulders will affect the movement of the pelvis. The swinging of the arms in walking will liberate movement in the legs and pelvis. Balance in the pelvis cannot be achieved without balance in the rest of the body.

Knowledge of the pelvic anatomy is absolutely necessary before doing any intimate work in the area. It is preferable for a body worker to have done some dissections or at least to have observed some dissections previously. There are only a few areas where damage can be done from ignorance. Knowing these areas is essential.

In order to do detailed pelvic work, it is vital that the practitioner be comfortable with his or her own pelvis. In general, any part of our own bodies that we don't want touched will create problems in our work. There is the tendency either to avoid that area in others or conversely to work too roughly there. I have had many a massage where my abdomen was not even touched, much less the pubic region.

This inhibition is especially true in touching the pelvic area. Any tentativeness can result in confusion on the part of the receiver. The element of shame could arise, or the client may misinterpret the touch as provocatively sensual, sexual, or even a sexual come-on. There must be an awareness of any sexual attraction to the client. A message of sexual interest can definitely be relayed by "sexual touch."

Sexual touch can be conveyed in touching any part of the body. It can be demonstrated by practicing with a friend. Put your hands on any part of the other person's body. First send "neutral" energy through your hands. Without moving, put sexual intention into your touch. I did this once in a rather large workshop of body workers. The "practitioner" was standing behind the "client" with hands on the shoulders. It happened that the men were paired with men and the women with women. I had them experience a number of different attitudes with their touch, ending with the sexual intention. People dropped their hands as though they had had an electric shock! There is also sexual reception on the part of the client. This is something of which a practitioner must have an awareness, and be able to counteract with an absolutely neutral touch.

I have given a number of workshops on the pelvis. I have always stressed: "If you don't feel comfortable around the anus or the groin, don't work there." It will create nothing but confusion and have an adverse effect on the results of the work. I suggest that the body worker practice first with a friend.

The best effect of the work is to make use of the client's breathing and as much movement as is appropriate. The full exhale is emphasized. When an area is touchy or painful, the tendency is to gasp and hold the breath on the inhale, which tightens the tissue. The exhale is the relaxing part of the breath. All good athletic trainers are aware of the importance of breathing into and through the touchy parts to the relaxing exhale. Exhale on flexion. Inhale on extension.

Working on the buttocks, the relationship to other parts of the body should be considered. It is an advantage to lengthen the long muscles of the back all the way down to the coccyx. Attention to the tightness in the lower back, the lumbar region, is necessary to reverse the effect of its pulling up on the pelvic bone. Ideally the lower back will respond to the breath, lengthening with the inhale and relaxing with the exhale. When this occurs, the buttocks can be more relaxed.

Hamstrings in men are generally short and tight. This relates to the narrower pelvis of the male. They can be liberated by a "lifting" of the muscles from the underlying tissue. There are two aspects of the stickiness of the hamstrings. One is the outer margins where the fascia glues them down to the adductor magnus underneath. The other is the fascia binding the lateral and medial hamstrings together. This requires the intention of separation of the muscles from each other. The most merciful way to do this is to have the client lie on his stomach, bending his leg at the knee. During this movement, the aberrant effect of the inner adductors and the outer iliotibial tract can be observed and addressed. The lengthening of the hamstrings will relieve the pull down on the lower margin of the gluteus maximus and the tuberosities (Fig. 14-1).

The approach to a "tight ass" proceeds more smoothly with a balance of education, sensitivity, and humor. One way to initiate awareness of the region is to have the client deliberately tighten his anus and then let it go. People are not aware of tightness in an area when the tightness is always there. When the anus is squeezed to the extreme, one can observe how the entire perineum is drawn in and how the gluteus maximus muscles are drawn together. Upon relaxation of the anal sphincters, the space between the rami is usually wider than it was before the exercise began.

The texture of the buttocks can vary from being hard like iron to being very spongy. In those men who have a degree of lordosis and the butt sticks out in back (considered sexy by many), the more superficial gluteus maximus is usually very rigid and resistant. In men where the buttocks is like dough, the tight cords of the deeper lateral rotators can be palpated underneath.

In either case, the first chore is to lengthen the gluteus maximus and

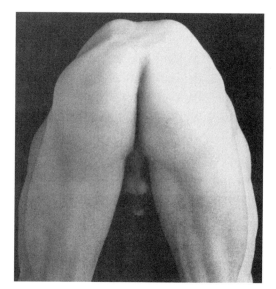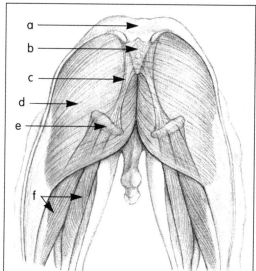

FIGURE 14-1

Relationship of hamstring muscles to gluteal region
(a) sacrum (b) coccyx (c) sacrotubrous lig. (d) gluteus maximus m. (e) ischial
tuberosity (f) hamstring m.

its fascia. It must be remembered that the upper border of the maximus
is usually glued down to the gluteus medius, which it overlaps. This border of stuck fascia may be so strong that it feels like a tendon. It will prevent the maximus from freely sliding over the medius. It should also be
remembered that its function goes down below the knee via the iliotibial
tract. Above, the fascia of the gluteus maximus is continuous with that of
the latissimus dorsi on the opposite side (Fig. 14-2).

The lower border of the maximus is attached to the coccyx, travels
across the ischial tuberosities and upper part of the hamstrings, and angles
down by the tract (ITT) to the knee. Since the coccyx frequently is pushed
deep and off to one side, the border of the maximus in that area will be
pulled deep with it. This lower border is then wrapped around the sacrotubrous ligament which angles from the sacrum to the ischial tuberosities and which is so strong that it can be considered part of the bony pelvis.
The ligament forms the border of the anal triangle (Fig. 14-3). The max-

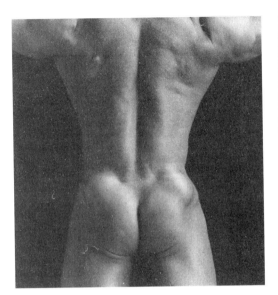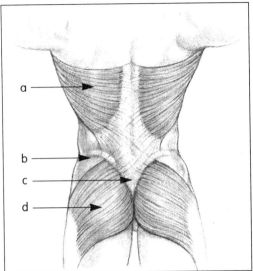

FIGURE 14-2
Fascial connections across the lumbar region
(a) latissimus dorsi (b) gluteus medius (c) sacrum (d) gluteus maximus

imus will often be stuck to the ischial tuberosities to the point that some books describe part of the maximus as coming from those bones. It will also stick to the upper portion of the hamstrings and effectively reduce their function. The project is to try to lift the maximus off these boundaries and allow it to lengthen.

The seven lateral rotators lie under the gluteus maximus. Sometimes there is a heavy fat pad which separates these two layers of muscle. Since the rotators attach to the posterior border of the greater tuberosities of the femur, their action when contracted is to rotate the femur backward. With chronic contraction, permanent depressions are created on the sides of the buttocks. This will relate to a narrow space between the ischial tuberosities.

Two of the rotator muscles have their upper attachments inside the pelvis. The piriformis is attached to the underside of the sacrum, while the body of the obturator internus lies inside the lower pelvic bowl. Their usual contraction may cause the space between the femur and the bony pelvis to be practically non-palpable. An effective approach is to work in

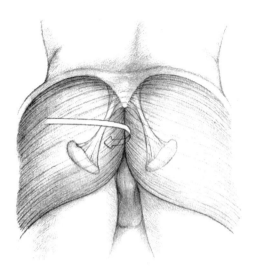
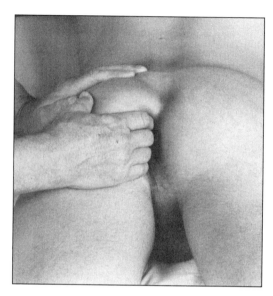

FIGURE 14-3
Lifting gluteus maximus off sacrotubrous ligament
(arrow indicates direction of work away from anus)

the area between the femur and the pelvic bone while the client is rotating the leg in and out in the hip joint (Fig. 14-4).

The piriformis is usually involved in the pain of sciatica. (Piriformis spasm and pain without the sciatic effect is a different matter and yet treatable in a similar fashion.) The piriformis muscle may lie over the nerve, under the nerve, or be bisected by the nerve. It is profitable to work both ends of the muscle attachment—the femur and the sacrum. The heavy pad over the sacrum, especially at the sacroiliac junction, needs attention and softening. The junction is classified as being slightly movable and most often is not movable at all because of the padding.

It is effective to free the coccyx and its ligaments as much as possible by working on either side of the bone focusing on the base next to the sacrum. This can be extremely uncomfortable and the touch must be modified accordingly. Obviously, care must be taken not to injure the bone, which lies at the top of the inverted V created by the ligaments (Fig. 14-3). The coccyx is frequently bent to one side or the other. This seems to act like a hook of the fascia extending down into the leg. The coccyx is actually a series of four little vertebrae. There are Rolfing class stories of a client breaking a stick or pencil while the Rolfer was working around the coccyx. No heart attacks have been reported, but skipped heartbeats and flushing of the Rolfer has been noted.

On the side, the action of the gluteus medius is a factor in pelvic tightness. This muscle extends from the outer border of the ilium to the upper border of the femur. Chronic contraction will in effect jam the femur up into the joint and restrict the movement. Since the fascia of the medius is continuous with that of the abdominal oblique muscles, shortening will contribute to the "love handles." These "handles" are not as much fat as people think.

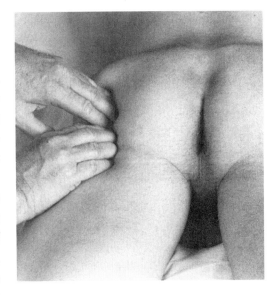

FIGURE 14-4
Working the area between the femur and the pelvic bone

An effective way to lengthen the medius is to press downward on the top of the femur while the client is on his side, flexing and extending at the hip joint. The majority of my clients had more of a waistline after ten sessions of Rolfing—without losing weight.

In the front, there may be a heavy fat pad covering the pubic bone. Since this is the area of the suspensory ligaments of the penis, the pad will not allow the penis to come to its full visual extension. What we usually feel of the bone through the pad is the tip only. The body of the pubic symphysis angles down. To truly affect the pad, one must pull down the penis to "scoop" up the tissue headward. To accomplish this maneuver, the client must have developed trust, the practitioner must be comfortable touching the penis even through cloth, and an explanation of why this is being done is more than helpful. Making this pubic pad more elastic will lessen the pulling in of the penis by the levator ani and decrease a pull upward by the rectus abdominus (Fig. 14-5).

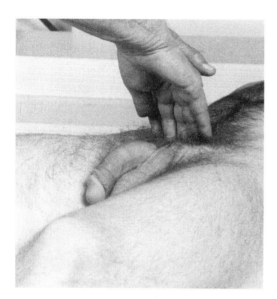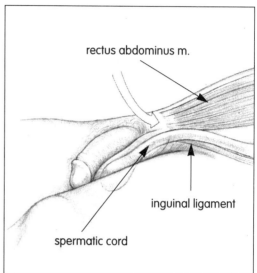

FIGURE 14-5
Lifting pad off pubic bone
(arrow indicates direction of work on pubic bone)

The inguinal region is the area where care must be taken. Anatomical knowledge is essential. The inguinal ligament angles from the edge of the pubic prominence to the anterior superior spines (ASS) of the ilium. These are the bony points that are very prominent in thin people. The ligament may actually be a number of ligaments running parallel to each other. This will vary depending on how the person has used his body. The ligament is formed by the joining of the bottom borders of the internal and external abdominal oblique muscles.

The spermatic cord starts about midway between the pubic bone and the ASS. It lies in the inguinal canal, just above the ligament. The inner ring of the canal is the place where the cord exits the body cavity and is the "weak" place where inguinal hernias can occur. The outer ring where the spermatic cord exits the canal lies at the edge of the pubic eminence. It is here where the spermatic cord becomes palpable as it descends down into the scrotum.

The fragility of the tissue at the internal ring can result in an opening

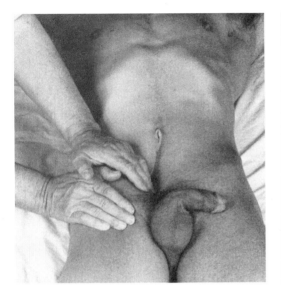 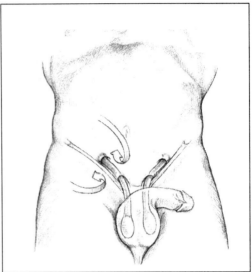

FIGURE 14-6
Lifting the spermatic cord and inguinal ligament
(arrows indicate direction of lift)

of the canal into which intestine can protrude and herniate. Dr. Ida Rolf stated that if an area is too weak, a compensatory area must be too strong. The psoas crosses the pubic bone just inside the anterior superior spines, where it often seems to be stuck to the bone. This can exert a lateral pull on the internal inguinal ring, spreading it. Tight abdominal muscles may pull on the ring from above and tight adductors can pull the ring down from below.

It is safe to work on the psoas from the side since the spermatic cord extends only halfway from the pubic eminence to the anterior superior spines. It is also safe to work above and below the inguinal ligament, avoiding the nerves and blood vessels in the femoral triangle. The artery in the triangle can be sensed easily by its pulsation, and obviously one must not press down directly on top of it. Any work in this area should be toward the spermatic cord—not pulling away from it in any way. It can be visualized as a gentle lifting of the ligament and cord from the tissue underneath (Fig. 14-6).

There exists in the body a spiral twist which has been termed by osteopaths as the common compensatory pattern. Part of this spiral is a structural shift of the left hip to the side. This exerts a strong pull from the base of the penis on the left side, seeming to go underneath the inguinal ligament, to the left margin of the ilium. The pull results in a toughening of the tissue in that area. The penis will be pulled to the left. The left descending spermatic cord feels glued to that side of the penis. It is estimated that 75% of men "hang to the left" (Fig. 7-9). Even those men whose penis points to the right seem to have a tightening at the base of the left side of the penis. The pattern does not seem to differ in men born south of the equator, which I noted when I was Rolfing in Brazil and Australia (an attempt at a joke referring to the water going down the drain in a different direction south of the Equator!).

The strong left pull on the penis can be modified by working gently between the spermatic cord and the base of the penis on that side. Here anatomical knowledge is again essential, as is comfort with touching the area. The left ischiocavernosus muscle at the base of the penis can be palpated and separated from the cord. The continuation of the tough tissue under the inguinal ligament can be lengthened by working underneath the ligament from above with a scooping action (Fig. 14-7).

Often the perineum (urogenital diaphragm) between the rami will be very narrow in men. The tissue can feel like cement. This is an extremely touchy area. It is possible to work on the bony surface by directing the client to feel the breath in the "bottom" of the abdomen. When both the client and practitioner are at ease with each other, space can be created by putting the fingers in the 'V' of the rami and waiting for some release with the exhale.

Sometimes working around the base of the penis and on the perineum will result in an enlargement of the penis. When this happens, the men are obviously very pleased. This increase in size is not surprising when one realizes that a percentage of the penis lies inside the perineum. If the inward pull on the penis is relaxed, more of it can appear on the surface. This does not always happen, so it is hardly something that we can put in our advertisements! It seems that some men are successful in letting go of muscular clenching and others are not.

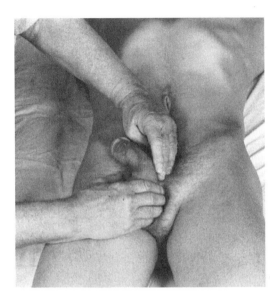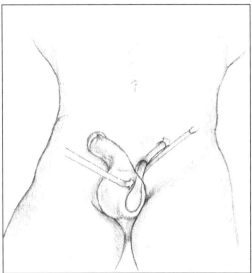

FIGURE 14-7
Separating left spermatic cord from base of penis
(arrow indicates direction of loosening of left spermatic cord from base of penis)

Under normal circumstances, the penis is not addressed in body work in general. On rare occasions, a situation occurs where this can be considered. If we view the penis as consisting of highly vascularized fascia, the thought of working on it is not that extreme. It should be emphasized to the client that manipulation of the penis is not part of Rolfing. An agreement must be reached between Rolfer and client before such work is undertaken.

One time a client came to me with a pronounced local swelling on the left side of his penis under the glans or head. He was experiencing extreme pain at the base of his penis on the left side. The pain was causing multiple erections which were sexual in feeling. Temporary relief was obtained by ejaculation. The relief was not long-lasting. On palpation, I found a cord-like structure about the size of the lead in a pencil extending down the left side of the penis (starting at the swelling), across the left side of the perineum, and seeming to end at the left side of the anal sphincter, which was tight. I manipulated down the cord on the left side of the penis, followed it across the perineum, and in the anal area I superficially endeavored to relax the anal sphincter on the left side. After three sessions of this work, the swelling, pain, and local tightness were gone. The client had experienced the Rolfing series previously. This allowed him to be responsive to such subtle work.

Another client came to me from another Rolfer with the complaint that his penis had been "broken" during sexual intercourse. This accident had caused a tough thickening midway in the penis. He said that when he was erect, the penis bent sharply at that area, making intercourse difficult and painful. I worked on his penis several times after explaining that this was not Rolfing. Since he did not get aroused during the sessions, I was not able to observe the bending of the penis which he described. The tight area softened a little, his penis got thicker (from his report), and the bend did not straighten out. The best of ideas don't always work.

15

Exercises, Images, and Response

THE USE OF THE WORD "EXERCISE" generally indicates physical effort done to improve health, lose weight, or tone the body in general. There are other uses of the word. We can exercise our minds or our abilities to accomplish tasks of various types.

In this discussion, I am presenting the idea of the exercise of awareness, focusing on the pelvic region. There are a number of exercises that I suggest to attain or retain pelvic openness in men. These exercises require motivation and self-permission to feel in that area. Consulting some kind of movement or body therapist would be advisable to start.

There are so many taboos that can be involved. Feeling pleasure in your body in general is not considered manly in many cultures. The idea of using sexual energy for living can be new and intimidating. Sexual energy for something other than sex is a difficult concept for many men to accept. They have great resistance to talking about it. As I have talked to various men about this project, many have told me: "Women talk freely about their pelvis, we never do."

The exercises are based on sensing the breath down to the perineum. They involve both the inhale and the exhale. First is the awareness of the response to the breath in the man's abdominal region—how far down the movement goes and where it doesn't go. This can involve the use of a mirror, one's hand, or another person's hand. Generally the breath response in the abdomen stops somewhere around the belly button.

In order to begin to have the awareness of abdominal breath response, the man must change from a "doing" to an "allowing" attitude. Awareness is an exercise. Each shift in gravity, e. g. lying down, sitting, standing, will make a difference in the awareness. In any position, the ideal is for the man to feel the breath lift his body from the pelvic floor.

The easiest position is lying on the back. An image I often use is for the man to imagine that the breath is coming into his body via the perineum and then spreading like a 'V' up to his chest (armpits), with the exhale going back out of the perineum. This is difficult for some men. The idea of anything pleasurable near their anus is too threatening. There is also the concern of passing gas.

An alternative is to imagine that on the inhale the breath comes into the umbilicus, going up to the chest and down to the crotch simultaneously and coming back out of the umbilicus with the exhale. This is much easier for many men. If they feel no response at all, I suggest that they pretend that they feel the perineal area with the breath. This pretense surprisingly can bring the breath response that far down in the body, although they may not feel it at the time.

If the man brings his knees up to his chest while lying down, the perineum (to varying degrees) will open and make it easier to feel the breath in that area. The ischial tuberosities can actually widen. To some it is much too uncomfortable to have the feeling of vulnerability of the anus. One man said he had not been in that position since he was a baby. (Another position is to be on one's knees and elbows with the butt raised to open and to allow breath into the perineal area. This again may be too threatening.)

While a man is on his back, he can practice a "pelvic rock." This is a very gentle rocking of the lower pelvis using the lower rectus abdominus to gently pull up the pubic bone. The idea is to do this rock without clenching the butt muscles. This motion differs from a "pelvic lift," which uses the legs and raises the lower back as well as the buttocks. The pelvic rock usually requires some guidance at first. It is not usual for a man to feel the movement that low. When I mention that this might improve one's sex life, there is frequently a more enthused response. I once did a workshop where I had a room full of straight and gay men thoroughly enjoying the rocking of their pelvis.

A way for a man to become aware of the anoperineal area is to use contract/release of the muscles in that region. A man usually has a tight ass of which he is not aware. He can't release what feels normal. If he contracts the anal sphincters to the fullest extent and then releases the muscles, he may feel the difference. Since the anal sphincters are attached to the perineal and penis muscles, that area will also be contracted and released. With some sophistication, the contraction of the perineal muscles separate from that of the anal muscles can be effected. While this feeling of the muscle action is easier in the lying-down position, it can be used in any position.

As men grow older, there can be less tone in the anal and/or perineal muscles. Without practice, they can become flabby like other muscles not used. This lack of tone can be a factor in urinary incontinence or a less than satisfactory erection. The contractions described above are similar to the Kegel exercises for women, developed for urinary incontinence and/or tightening the muscles of the vagina. These contractions involve the same muscles present in men—muscles at the base of the penis, the perineal muscles, the anal sphincters, and the pelvic diaphragm. The instructions for women involve tightening these muscles twenty times, several times a day. It couldn't hurt men to get more tone in that area. It's an exercise that can be practiced in public without notice.

There are two problems that can be modified by more awareness and better tone of the urogenital musculature. These are the muscles that squeeze out the last drops of urine at the end of urination. Particularly in older men, there is a residue of urine remaining in the urethra which drips out after the penis is put back into pants or underwear. I see yellow stains, however in the underwear of men of all ages when they come for bodywork. Stronger muscle tone in the perineal region can help the last shaking to be more effective.

The opposite problem is that of "pee-shyness." In this case the muscles are overly contracted and inhibit the opening of the urethra at the base of the penis to allow the free flow of urine. Using the breath to relax these muscles can help to overcome the embarrassing problem.

As mentioned, the pelvis in men is normally more narrow than in women. This narrowness is compounded by the habitual holding and tightening of the perineal/anal region, resulting in a restriction of movement. A way to widen a narrow perineum is to sit on a tennis ball. If the ball is placed in the space between the 'V' of the bony rami, it will certainly bring awareness to the area. If the ball is centered, it can be very painful because the body weight will be centered on the base of the penis. Preferably the ball can be placed under the ischial tuberosities, one at a time. This is the area where the hamstrings are attached to the tuberosities. The idea is not to roll back and forth, but to rest on the spot for ten full cycles of breathing. This can allow release to happen, rather than trying to force it

In order to sit, most men clench their buttocks and come down on tight muscle. Since this is uncomfortable, the tendency is to slouch backward and sit almost on their lower spines. Most furniture does not encourage sitting upright without effort. Sitting upright with more ease can be achieved by finding the bony platform between the legs—the 'V'-shaped bone between the base of the penis and the anus. The easiest way is to spread the buttocks with the hands either in the process of or after sitting. This can be done at home—probably not in public. I had to do this spreading at home for some time before I was O.K. with the feeling of sitting on my anus.

A way of discouraging the butt-clenching habit in public sitting is for the man to bend his knees to the appropriate height of the chair and then "point" his anus to the junction between the bench and the back of the chair (legs spread for balance). Often he may feel as though he is sticking his buttocks out and looking silly. Checking this gesture in the mirror is helpful. It never looks as silly as it feels at first. If he feels the bony points of the tuberosities, he is sitting too far back. He needs to lean more forward on the bones, which is a difficult concept at first. It is totally contrary to his usual habit of sitting. It will change the way he presents himself, which may be uncomfortable at first. The hope is that the man feels that balance and breath are holding him up, not muscle. Practically, when sitting for a long period of time, the more upright position is much easier on the lower back.

Several years ago, I was visiting a friend in the wine country of California. We went to a restaurant I'd been to once many years before. I was very surprised when the owner recognized me. He said he recognized the way I was sitting. He said: "I've never seen anyone sit as straight as you do." I had been totally unconscious of the way I was sitting.

Feeling the breath down into the pelvis is the most difficult when standing. This can be helped by the man doing a pelvic rock. It is easier to learn with assistance of another pair of hands. With the man's knees slightly bent, the other person places his/her fingers on the coccyx and pubic eminence (it probably should be a good friend). This describes the sling of the pelvic diaphragm or pelvic floor connecting the two points. The idea is to see if he can feel the subtle rocking of that sling. It is not a movement of the lower back thrusting the pelvis forward and back. The movement is much lower and more gentle. One can think of the pelvis like a baby cradle. It can rock on the heads of the femurs. If he can become aware of this rocking, he can use the rocking of the pelvis in walking—not doing it—feeling it in movement. To consciously *do* the rock results in a jerky, stilted gait; to *allow* the movement and to *feel* it results in a more graceful flow through the pelvis.

Allowing the breath down to the pelvis is important in walking. It contributes to a smooth and flexible stride. For men with chronic back pain, the tendency in starting movement is to "grab" with the muscles of the lower back, blocking the movement of the pelvis as well as the lower back. It is a "normal" protective response. This is especially true in running, where there is the fear of falling. This limiting of the breath to the upper body is much like the cold-water gasp. The walking becomes stiff with no movement through the pelvis since the pelvis is being held rigid by the spastic back muscles. It takes considerable patience and trust on the part of the man to allow a deep and full breath to go to the lower back. The contraction of the muscles in the back only increases the discomfort. The deeper breathing with good exhales will allow for the relaxation of the back muscles and subsequent movement of the lower back and pelvis.

Similar relationships between muscle spasms, holding of the breath, and lack of flow of movement through the pelvis can be present with spasms of the abdomen, sides, and even the ribs. Other parts of the body are obviously affected in movement under these conditions. All seem to have an effect on the working relationship between the trunk and the legs, and all are affected by the breathing.

Another consideration in walking is the frequent tendency to "walk around" the genitals. In other words, the genitals are quiet while the rest of the body is in movement. This produces an awkward gait of the legs swinging around the genitals. An exercise is to feel the genitals swinging with movement, walking "through" them. It can be helpful for the man to feel as though weights are hanging from the genitalia. Observations of the movement in a mirror can be used to initiate awareness.

The sensual aspects of this awareness are especially important. Sensual feelings can be a part of sex for a man—opinion seems to say otherwise for many. Many men are not terribly interested in any feelings in sex except for the penis. Sensory feelings in the anal/genital region can be stimulated by gentle self-massage. It is almost the opposite of masturbation. There is the requirement for permission to feel pleasure in the groin, perineal, and buttocks region. The man's hands and breath can be used to experience enjoyment. Sensual massage will allow the man to enjoy the pleasant feeling without expectation of performance.

A suggestion I frequently make to men while working in the pubic area is to imagine that their penis is like the handle of a torch. The fire goes up inside. Men are trained to prevent fluids from leaking out of the penis at inappropriate times. This can result in a habitual pulling in of the structure for constant control. The idea of something going into the body via the penis gives a different response, a letting go. Many men come back and tell me how much they enjoy their "handle." Sensations there in everyday life are a new experience.

To some men, this analogy means nothing in terms of feeling. There is no interest in any fire inside them. A picture they sometimes relate to better is that of the base of the penis being like a hook which pulls the body down. Some men relate more to a feeling while others prefer a more mechanical image.

As a result of pelvic work and/or awareness, men have reported a feeling of more energy. (It must be emphasized that the pelvis is not the only part of a man's body in which feeling has been liberated, and yet it is the most provocative.) The response to more openness is evident by bigger smiles and a sense of less tension.

Other benefits that have been reported:

- more openness in personal and professional relationships.
- enjoyment of sensual feelings.
- more enjoyable sexual activity.
- more complete body orgasms.
- relief of elimination problems.
- clearer relations with both men and women.
- enjoyment of the idea of using sexual energy for creation of all kinds, not just recreational and procreational.

Obviously, it is much too naive to say that freeing up the pelvis will totally change a person's outlook on life. It certainly does give life more sparkle. Since the body is a total unit, ease of movement and more openness of feelings in one area will affect the entire body.

When little boys can cry, we will have achieved much in men's relationships.

16

Masturbation

EVERY MAN DOES IT; no man will talk about it; almost every man will deny it; usually there is guilt associated with it; frequently it is done in haste to get it over with. This is one of men's darkest secrets, especially adult men, and most especially men in a relationship—married or otherwise committed.

A baby boy will instinctively reach for his penis. It is his first toy, the touch of which brings pleasure. Often this gesture results in the adult response of "no, no." This could start the awareness that this is something that must be touched in secret.

Toilet training can be the next input of negative attitudes about the penis. This can be especially true if the boy is trained at an early age. The penis can become an embarrassing part of his body.

As boys go through their early stages of growing up, there is often groping of the genitals in public. This continues into manhood in many cultures. Could this be a checking to determine that they are still there, or could it be a sign of manhood? The amount of material in the grope may indicate the size of the genitals.

When does "playing with the penis" become masturbation? In the past, the idea seemed to be that it was masturbation when ejaculation started. It has now been shown that puberty or interest in sex starts long before the physical signs are evidenced. Maybe it's masturbation when one starts pumping up and down.

One man told me that he had started "masturbating" at about the age of seven years. An older cousin, who did ejaculate, taught him how to jerk his penis up and down. It felt good and he continued to do this; at about the age of twelve, something white shot out and he discovered the real pleasure of orgasm. He proudly demonstrated this phenomenon to his friends, who were slower in development. His mother was a very strong Christian and became suspicious of his behavior. Hasty jerking off and subsequent guilt became the pattern that persisted for much of his life.

When I was younger, I assumed that men who were married never had to masturbate again. Since this was such an unspoken subject, it was years before I learned that I was not the only one who thought this.... When I was writing this book, I discovered that marriage or a committed relationship, straight or gay, is not the end of masturbation. Under the cover of "scientific interview" men were quick to assure me that self-satisfaction continued to be necessary and/or desirable.

My specialty over twenty-five years of Rolfing has been working on the pelvis. Since Rolfing is based on the idea of the whole body, it seemed that the penis must be part of that whole. I talked to men about relaxing at the time of orgasm to allow the pleasure in their entire body rather than limiting it to the penis. I suggested that they try this by themselves when they did not feel the need to satisfy someone else. I was amazed at how many men of all ages were delighted to have permission to masturbate. In general they came back with big smiles.

A big difference in attitude is the idea of making love to yourself. The early pattern is to beat-off quickly to get the relief and release. This can transfer into your adult sexual behavior—get hard, get off, and go to sleep. Not many men take the time to enjoy the feeling of an erection in and of itself. Even stroking the penis when it is soft can be enjoyable when there is no judgment involved. In fact, the penis is more sensitive when it is not completely hard.

Making love to yourself obviously takes time. It's like having sex with another person—sometimes there can be time for extensive love-making and other times a "quickie" has to do. I have seen married men at the train station, coming into the men's room from their morning commute;

they walk up to a urinal, stroke their penis quickly, ejaculate into the urinal, wipe the penis with a tissue, and go on about their day. They show about as much emotion as if they were urinating. Obviously in this situation, orgasm is not a factor.

The way in which men masturbate differs. Men who are not circumcised have more foreskin to play with—more to rub up and down. Circumcised men seem to be more sensitive at the base of the glans almost from the beginning of foreplay. When the glans emerges from the prepuce in uncircumcised men, the base of the glans is then extremely sensitive. Thus, the stroke will differ from man to man.

Some men will grip their penis with the four fingers, the thumb out at an angle, rubbing the entire body of the penis up and down. Another pattern is the use of the thumb and first finger, focusing more on the area under the head of the penis; in this case, the other three fingers are held out to the side. There are many variations. It seems probable that a man will hold his penis in much the same way when he urinates.

It is not unusual for a man to be one-handed when he masturbates—right or left. There have been times when as I worked on one hand of a man, his penis became erect. A few men were cool enough to mention that this was the hand used for masturbation.

Men differ greatly in the amount of pre-cum. Pre-cum is a clear liquid which oozes from the penis before ejaculation. It can be somewhat independent of active sexual behavior. In some cases, just the thought of sex may induce the emission of pre-cum. I have had several clients who became semi-erect when I worked on their pubic bone. The pre-cum leaked out of their penis like a faucet and, yet, they seemed to have no awareness of this. Other men basically have no pre-cum at all. It would seem that the more pre-cum, the less need for external lubrication. Some men like it dry, others like it slippery.

Making love to yourself means more than "beating your meat." A common practice is to place the alternate hand behind the testicles and press on the muscles at the base of the penis and the external sphincter muscle of the anus. This increases the hardness of the erection and indirectly stimulates the prostate. An additional stimulation is to put a finger into the anus. "Making love" is really just taking the time to stroke and stimulate yourself on any part of your body in relation to the masturbation.

Is the secret around masturbation the result of fear of being less secure about your sexual image if you have to satisfy yourself? Or is it a sign that your sexual relationships must be less than satisfactory? Many partners, male and female, feel angry or inadequate if the man confesses to or is found out to masturbate. With the current increase in men's groups, the secret may become more accepted.

Such total acceptance will not come soon, if ever. There are many cultural and religious attitudes against masturbation (for example, see Appendix III). At present, progress is made if individual men become more accepting of doing what comes naturally.

17

Male Sexuality

THERE IS THE OLD SAYING that the size of a man's car is inversely proportional to the size of his penis. I have heard many women say that men's brains are in their penis. It seems probable that in many cases, emotions and sensations are localized there. I have mentioned this to a number of men. Without exception they have agreed that their penis does govern their lives—some agree at once, usually with a laugh—some grudgingly agree—other strongly disagree, only to tell me later, rather sheepishly, that this was true.

One definition I have heard for sex is that it consists of the interaction between holes and poles; expanding this, it also could be the interaction between poles and poles or holes and holes. Men's approach to sex seems to fall in four categories:

- Anonymous sex: no personal communication, just the physical act.
- Casual sex: a pickup, some conversation, sex on the first meeting.
- Dating: several meetings before sex, getting to know the person first.
- Nesting: every man or woman is analyzed as a potential committed relationship.

These categories apply to both straight and gay men. Some men are stuck in one classification. Others will vary depending on the circumstances. The eternal problem with any classification is that it can't fit everyone all of the time.

The penis is the structure that allows men to feel unique. Throughout our lives it has been the basis of envy, guilt, shame, pride, embarrassment, pain, concern, passion, pleasure, and ecstasy. It can be a "magic wand" to demonstrate love or it may be a weapon to express anger. Men often look at it as a separate entity, giving it a name. The penis can be either a fun toy or a bothersome appendage viewed with disgust or discomfort. It can be used to increase self-esteem or to temporarily numb negative feelings. It can be isolated emotionally from the rest of the body. Often it is used as a tool to prove manliness.

Some men have a penis so fickle that it requires a frequent change of partners. This is true for both gay and straight men. For some men, using their penis (or using another's) is the only way they can feel of any value. The "sexual athlete" occurs in both populations.

A variation is the man who requires sex with his partner every time they are together. A friend of mine told me that her husband has insisted on sex every night they've been together for almost thirty years. Her comment was: "How many orgasms can a woman have?" She must not mind altogether since, in the company of close friends, she will tease her husband about the size of his penis. Her husband is the type of man who is serious about everything he does. He may believe that this is what married people must do. . . . At any rate, it seems to work since they are very affectionate.

Another friend of mine was upset because his boyfriend did not want to have sex every time they were together. The boyfriend would sometimes like just to cuddle together. It is interesting that my friend, who is a very talented man, will brag about himself only in regard to his sexual ability. He is very modest about his other accomplishments.

An older male friend was dating a much younger man who turned out to be a total "top" sexually. The younger man insisted on sex each time they were together and the scenario was the same. There were a few kisses followed by the younger man requiring oral and/or anal sex. There was no attempt to sexually stimulate the older man. At first, the older man was complimented by the attention of a young stud and submitted to this for some time, loving the kisses and enduring the sex. He finally insisted that the young man stroke his lower body and penis in a sensual way to turn him on. The young man seemed to have no experience or interest in this kind of "love-making." His touch was awkward and rough. Finally they both agreed that they were sexually incompatible. When the older man told this story to his female friends, they said that this was not unusual in their sexual experience with men.

On the other hand, one-night stands can be the rule; a greater number of conquests can be made in a shorter period of time. With some of these men there is the need for instant gratification. With others, there is the pride in how long they can maintain an erection with a different partner. This may indicate the need to keep the ego inflated and to cover feelings of inadequacy. These athletes are extremely proud of their proficiency in seduction. The cruising is constant, always on the lookout for "fresh meat." They may infer that it is not their fault that so many men, women, or both are attracted to them. It is their "duty" to satisfy as many as they can. It's a game: "How much and how often can I score." Actually, it may be a case of hiding other emotions through sexual activity.

Spending an evening socially with one of these sexual athletes, either straight or gay, can end in frustration for the companion. When the potential quarry is spotted, there is an abrupt character change. The attention shifts, often to the point that the companion is ignored and frequently dumped without a thought.

Some men function well sexually only in orgies. This gives them permission to give and receive as much anonymous touching as they want. It is touching without the fear of emotional involvement. It is not unusual for orgies to be conducted in the dark. Without emotional involvement and visual input, the erogenous zones can be stimulated and explored without fear of judgment.

With some men, sexual desire can be insatiable. There are more and more meetings for those who suffer from sexual addiction. Based on the "12-Step" programs pioneered by Alcoholics Anonymous, these meetings attempt to help the sexual addict identify and recover from destructive patterns of behavior.

Active promiscuity is considered to be a sign of immaturity by many people. It's like the little boy who says, "I want, I want, I want." Any emotions are kept superficial. Deeper feelings would give a sense of vulnerability and intimacy, which is uncomfortable and intimidating. Those who actively pursue multiple sex partners may be very proficient in the casual pickup, thereby enhancing their ego. Or they may play it safe emotionally by frequenting prostitutes or hustlers. These types often are not good lovers since their attention is strictly on their own gratification and performance. I have received many comments that some men kiss around the face and neck just long enough to get below the waist and down to business: primarily to the serious business of intercourse. Penetration, in this case, is the name of the game. Then, getting off and getting gone!

Men can be sexual addicts without being actively sexual. Sex is almost constantly in such men's thoughts, and for many reasons (morals, culture, environment) they don't act it out. Some men live with very vivid sexual fantasies which may have started when they were young. The problem which arises is that the occasional sexual encounter is seldom as exciting as it is in their imagination. Other men may become voyeurs—getting their kicks by watching others. There can be the excessive use of pornography for sexual release. Or they may become extreme moralists condemning others who do what they would secretly like to do.

I have heard older men asked by younger ones if the thoughts of sex diminish with age. Frequently the response is that they think more about it, because they are doing less of it.

It often seems that men tend to focus on parts of the body, rather than the whole person. Straight men may have a preference for breasts or hips or legs or hair. Gay men often comment on asses, muscular development, crotches, or facial hair. I have often heard women say that they they are more concerned about the man's sensitivity than about how he looks. Men seem to focus much more on physical appearance. Often they seem not to care too much about what's inside as long as the packaging turns them on. What stimulates feeling in the penis is often given priority.

There are artificial solutions to sexual problems or feelings. Alcohol in small amounts tends to relieve inhibitions. Too much and the penis loses its potency. With marijuana, there are individual responses. Some people are very turned on while others become withdrawn. Drugs such as cocaine initially will stimulate sexual interest and performance. Taken in quantity or on a habitual basis, it produces the "cocaine dick," which can be very limp and nonfunctional. This is an attempt to use chemical substances to subdue innate feelings and to produce an artificial stimulus. Other ways to cover sensitivity are excessive talking, role playing, acting out fantasies etc., etc.

Men are constantly searching for their lost youth and vibrant penis. Cosmetic surgery has become more accepted by men. One established method of feeling young has been to find younger companions/sex partners. This is another pattern that is true for both straight and gay men. When men change their partners, they usually end up with a younger one. Perhaps they think that the youth of their companion will revitalize their own bodies. There is the ego factor of being seen with a younger person. They do not realize that the physical contrast to a younger person makes them look older. It may also be assumed by others that there is some kind of financial arrangement involved.

The aspect of age is different in straight and gay cultures. Many young women are attracted to older men. It's not only the factor of a better financial situation, but women seem to enjoy the maturity and experience that come with years of living. In gay culture, youth is very much the focus. There is the saying, "There is nothing more useless than an old queen." The measures that older gay men resort to in an attempt to look younger can be unfortunate. Heavy makeup looks like heavy makeup. Face-lifts frequently look like an older man with a face-lift but without character. (This also applies to older male actors who have cosmetic surgery. Maybe this is to justify being paired with younger companions on the screen.) For the older gay men, especially in the larger cities, special programs are being developed to help them feel useful in this society.

There is a collection of quotes entitled What Women Say About Men. The majority of the quotes refer to the immaturity of men: men as overgrown boys. One from Françoise Sagan is: "I like men who behave like men—strong and childish." The aspect of strength has been emphasized lately with the increased interest in body building. The misconception is that strength and muscle bulk are synonymous. True strength comes from muscle tone, integrated body movement, and flexibility. The development of extreme muscle bulk will actually interfere with body movement. Large "traps, "delts," and "pecs" in the chest and shoulder will restrict the movement in the shoulder joint. I once saw a man whose shoulders were so overdeveloped that he could not bring a cup up to his mouth with his arm; he had to bring his head forward to it. Over-development of the thighs and "gluts" likewise will inhibit free movement in the hip joint. Such men walk like robots.

Working out to build tone is a good idea when not overdone, especially when combined with aerobics. Trainers have told me that working out three times a week is sufficient to build up muscle tone. The best idea might be to combine the workout with movement, such as Yoga or some of the Chinese techniques. Flow of movement on a daily basis is a concept which doesn't exist in most men's mentality.

Control is another factor that can rule a man's life and his relationships. Excessive control is often manifested by a lack of flexibility of attitudes. Overt actions are a way in which men fool themselves into believing that they are in control. The power game creates a competitiveness among men so that they can never be really close to each other. Being open and vulnerable is perceived as a dangerous exposure of one's self instead of an attribute of strength. Never ask for help—"I can do it myself!"

Many women have found that pretending to be passive is the best method of control. When men think they are in control, the woman usually can get what she wants. Men's egos must be massaged. The rise in the feminist movement has put a lot of straight men into a state of confusion. As women have become more assertive about their equal opportunity on the job and in the bedroom, these men cannot deal with their perceived loss of penis power.

Partly because of the confusion of the roles of men and women, men's groups have become more popular. Some groups focus on men reestablishing themselves as men, tough and rough. Other groups have emphasized men interacting with each other, building a trust between them, and becoming more sensitive to each other's needs. Building sensitive relationships with other men opens the way for them to experience their own feelings. This in turn allows men to become more sensitive to the needs of their partner, be it a man or a woman. The concept in groups is that as the man becomes more present, all of his relationships will improve.

A number of years ago, I was part of a men's group composed of straight and gay men. The prevailing complaint of all was the lack of a relationship. Week after week there was universal moaning about how to find a relationship. There do seem to be men who cannot function without a partner. I wonder if this need is real or is it conditioned by our family, friends, and culture? It seems as though a man might be able to be comfortable with his own company before embarking on a commitment to another man or woman.

A way in which a man can become more sensitive about the needs of others is to be more sensitive to his own need for touching. To do this, it seems imperative that the man become more aware of his own response to touch. If his own body does not respond to pleasant sensations, his attempt to please others becomes mechanical and artificial.

The opening up of sensitivity along with the freeing of body restrictions applies to more than sexual relationships. Friendships are also relationships which become enhanced in quality by more openness in mind, body, and spirit. Such openness can be stilted by fear of misinterpretation, e. g. the difference between intimacy and sexual come-on. One must be at ease with feelings of vulnerability, which are a part of the process. There is the constant fear of being rejected or being taken advantage of. Learning to trust in one's own feelings can be a guiding factor. First a person has to be aware of his internal emotions to be able to sense them. The courage to follow these "gut" feelings, and the ability to sense and trust them sooner, will develop and grow with practice.

I know two male friends who after many years of friendship decided to experiment sexually with each other. The sex was not especially rewarding and a distance developed between them. They avoided each other for many months. When they finally renewed communication, sex was not mentioned. Sex and friendship often do not mix.

When I used to give workshops about male sexuality, I would discuss some of the basis for homophobia. With straight men there are the fears that if they find another man attractive, they might be gay; if they have sexual activity once with a man, they might be gay; if they like touching another man, they might be gay. I mentioned these ideas to a group of gay men. They responded, "Don't you know that we have the same fears? If we find a woman attractive, we might be straight, etc." These workshops were more than twenty years ago. I wonder if those fears are as strong today. With the advent of AIDS, some gay men are getting married to women.

Using the terms "straight" and "gay" seems to allow for no levels of "gray." For example, there are many gay men who enjoy occasional sex with women. Many of them are even fathers whose sexuality does not affect their rapport with their children. On the other hand, there are straight men who are not adverse to a friendly blow-job or even more intimate contact with another man. In the latter case, alcohol is often the excuse "not to remember." The term "bisexual" is frowned upon by both straight and gay men as a cop-out. The general concept is that this is just hiding one's homosexuality. My sense is that we are all bisexual—which I have been told is a cliché.

For whom are these labels? Do we need to label ourselves for self-identity? Or are these labels for other people's convenience? I once heard a teacher being asked by a student if he was gay. The reply was: "I hate to be labeled for something I do so little of."

Achilles' heel might well be renamed "Achilles' penis." This is particularly evident for men in high profile positions or careers, be they entertainers, sports figures, or politicians. There are two sides to this conundrum. One aspect is the susceptibility of powerful or popular men to seduction by (usually) younger men or women for the purpose of their own self advancement. A modification of this is the "star fucker" whose intention is to add prominent names to his/her list of conquests.

The other side of the situation is the misuse of "penis power" by the more powerful man. Sexual harassment on the job is being reported more often. Yet the reports are not always taken seriously unless there are multiple incidents. The accusation of harassment can be misused. It may be real or it may be a retaliation for some resentment.

Inappropriate sexual activity, especially by politicians, has been great fodder for the media in recent times. It has ruined the careers of many men of intelligent and wise leadership potential. A President's penis brought about his impeachment and the near loss of his office!

18

Erectile Dysfunction (Impotence)

FOR CENTURIES, MEN HAVE BEEN LOOKING for the magic aphrodisiac that will bring the penis to a stronger and longer erection. Such items as certain bird feathers, snake oil, oysters, ginseng root, rhino horn, tiger penis, and yohimbine have been used with no or very limited success. Males can be easily fooled by placebo effect, which can temporarily ameliorate mild impotence. In the past, some doctors treated impotence with the male hormones (usually testosterone). This does not work, and there is the possibility that such treatment may increase the incidence of prostate cancer.

Types of cock rings have been used to maintain an erection. I know a man who used a metal cock ring for this reason. Unfortunately his erection was maintained—for days. It became unbearably painful. After several days he had to go to a doctor and have the ring filed off the base of his penis. The doctor's comment was, "I wonder how to describe this procedure in my records." The metal rings or too-tight rubber rings can cause injury to the blood vessels of the penis.

In this century, impotence was considered to be primarily "all in the head." Certainly performance anxiety can become a factor. After a few times of failure, the psychological effect can be self-reinforcing. There were those who believed that a non-functional penis was caused by "youthful follies." Since the 1980s, it has become more apparent that the problem is often more physical than psychological.

There are some estimates that a high percentage of men over forty have some problem with erectile dysfunction. Until recently, the majority of men were too embarrassed to see a physician about the problem. Those men who did seek treatment were greeted with rather unpleasant possibilities.

One was the use of an external vacuum pump. An erection was achieved by inserting the penis into the opening of the vacuum chamber and pumping until the penis hardened sufficiently. Once this was accomplished, a rubber ring was then slid off the pump onto the base of the penis to maintain the hard-on. This was less dangerous than a metal cock ring. The directions strongly stated that the erection should not be maintained for more than thirty minutes to avoid damage to the blood vessels. The rubber ring was then slid off the organ or cut off the base of the penis. This method was very cumbersome, uncomfortable, difficult to perform, and short-lived. There was the possibility of over-pumping and damaging the vasculature of the penis.

Another method was the injection of a solution into the corpora cavernosa of the penis with a hypodermic syringe. The solution contained a mixture of vasodilators. With the proper doses, this injection was successful in producing an erection which lasted from one to two hours. The negative side was that it was painful and the discomfort lasted long after the erection had subsided. There is also the mental consequence of sticking a needle into one's penis. In many ways, the end result was still worth it.

A far more drastic solution is the insertion of a penile implant. There are various types of implants. The simplest is the semirigid malleable implant placed in the underside of the penis. It provides a permanent erection and can be bent to fit into clothing. It is not great in a tight swim suit. More complicated are the inflatable implants that are placed in the corpora cavernosa. These are of varying degrees of complexity and generally will consist of two parallel hollow cylinders placed within the penis and a pump put in the scrotum (replacing one testicle). When desired, the hydraulic fluid in the pump can be squeezed up into the cylinders, producing an erection. This can be reversed by compressing the release valve on the side of the pump. Some men have been pleased with the result. It certainly is irreversible. The penises with implants that I have seen look somewhat abnormal and have a very rubbery feel to them.

A more appetizing method was the development of Muse®. A small pellet in a plastic syringe (no needle) was placed into the opening of the penis and "injected" in the penile cavity. The penis was then massaged to improve the absorption of the pill's contents into the penile tissue. The results with this method were mixed. There was some erectile reaction which did not seem to be sustained. This lasted a short period of time in popularity—in fact it did not become well known.

All of the above were eclipsed by Viagra®. This pharmaceutical compound has driven men almost into a frenzy. It has brought out the word "impotence" as a public term. Throughout the world, men's penises have quivered in anticipation of an erection on call. I have heard that Viagra® is selling on the black market at exorbitant prices. Men who are not impotent wanted more and stiffer. Older men left their wives or partners for better playgrounds. Urologists' offices became over-crowded.

Viagra® (as well as the injection methods) affects the blood supply to the penis. There is a chemical reaction which produces smooth muscle relaxation in the corpora cavernosa, allowing inflow of blood. Physicians say that Viagra® does not work unless the man is in a sexually stimulating situation (unlike the other stimulants). There are growing indications of adverse side effects. Any man with a heart problem should be very careful of the dosage.

Is this another sexual revolution for men? Although every man will suffer from "limp dick" occasionally, complete impotence has a devastating effect on a man's mental health. In these cases, Viagra® and like compounds may open a door some men had thought was closed forever. These are not the only men who are clamoring for the pill. Penis power may become stronger than ever.

19

Maturity

THERE ARE MANY WAYS to define maturity. Many women believe that men never reach maturity. They remain overgrown boys. Like boys, men certainly like their toys. For many straight men, there is the preoccupation with balls–tennis balls, golf balls, basketballs, footballs, volley balls, bowling ball, and other round toys. There is also the size and make of the car, the size of the barbecue, the size of the boat, and the price of the gardening and mechanical tools. This can be true for gay men also. Their toys can be extended to include sex toys–dildos, anal balls, and other kinky objects.

A simplistic way of looking at maturity can be body movement. Often it seems as though each joint has its own personality. A mature joint might be looked at as one that is freely mobile–being used in harmony with the rest of the body. Guarding (lack of movement) at one joint will affect the movement of all other joints.

Using this concept, an estimation of the degree of sexual maturity of the adult male can be defined by observing the freedom of movement of the pelvis. This will involve the movement of the pelvic bone (ilium) in the hip joint and the movement between the lumbar vertebrae and the sacrum. In the back, immobility will relate to the degree of tightness of the gluteal muscles and the rotators, protecting the anus. In the front, the muscle factors will be the lower abdominal muscles and the muscles of the upper thigh, pulling in the genitals. The combined tightness of these muscles produces the shortness in the groin area and the immovable dimples in the buttocks.

Relieving the pelvic protection first involves helping the man to become aware of the lack of movement and feeling. The use of the breath is a strong tool for this awareness (See Appendix II.) In general, people do not use the full breath, even in exercise. They do not completely exhale, leaving a residue of air in the lungs. The exhale is the relaxing part of the breath. Thus, without a complete exhale there is not the space for a full inhale.

With physical and/or emotional pain, the usual response is to hold the breath–taking very short breaths with little exhale. An example is jumping into cold water. The first response is to gasp. When a full breath is finally taken, the water is not so cold.

Once full breaths are achieved, the man's attention can then be directed to the area where the body does not respond to the breath. Most often the lack of response is in the pelvic bowl. Since the pelvic bowl is the bottom of the abdomen, it is possible to see and feel the breath response down that low.

Once the breathing response into the pelvis is achieved, movement of the pelvic area is available. The tight protective muscles can be manipulated. The client can become aware of the involuntary tightness and begin to let go in everyday life, letting it all hang out. It is necessary to be conscious of the fears and feelings of vulnerability that may arise from this feeling of freedom.

This is how the flow of movement through the pelvis can be considered a sign of a "mature" pelvis. Letting go of the penis and anus may be a big factor in letting go of the demons about sex. It can also be the beginning of allowing awareness to come to the surface.

Obviously, it is much too naive to say that freeing up the pelvis will totally change a person's outlook on life. It certainly does give life more sparkle. Since the body is a total unit, ease of movement and more openness of feelings in one area will affect the entire body.

When little boys can cry, we will have achieved much in men's relationships.

Rolfing

ROLFING IS THE MOST ESTABLISHED METHOD of Structural Integration or deep fascial manipulation. There are more than one thousand Rolfers practicing in twenty-seven countries, with about seven hundred in the United States.

Rolfing is a trademarked approach within the generic field of structural integration. It was developed by Ida P. Rolf, Ph.D., a biophysicist who earned her doctorate in the 1920s. She began doing her form of bodywork in the 1940s and 50s. Her clientele included Georgia O'Keefe and Buckminster Fuller, and she worked with other pioneers in the bodywork field. In the 1960s she began teaching at the Esalen Institute in California. She formed the Rolf Institute of Structural Integration in Boulder, Colorado, in 1972.

Rolfing involves a form of deep tissue work for reordering the body so as to bring its major segments—head, shoulders, thorax, pelvis, and legs—into a finer vertical alignment. The technique loosens or releases adhesions in the fascia, the flexible tissue that envelops our muscles and muscle groups. The fascia is supposed to move easily and allow easy articulation or movement of muscles or muscle groups past each other. However, trauma such as injury or chronic stress can cause stuck points or adhesions, in which the fascia is in a sense frozen, not allowing full freedom of movement.

The Rolfer works to restore this freedom of movement, resulting in a more balanced, vertical alignment of the body and often a lengthening or expansion of the body's trunk. Rolfing usually takes place over a series of ten organized sessions dealing with different areas of the body.

Breathing

I T IS COMMON IN BODYWORK to tell a client to "breathe into" an area. We do this as a way to help them become more aware of that area. It usually has to be explained that "a breath" means both inhale and exhale. In purely mechanical terms, breathing consists of the actions of the ribs and the diaphragm. During inhalation, the expansion of the ribs provides the chest breathing, while the diaphragm muscular flattening causes "abdominal breathing." Many people are either primarily chest or abdominal breathers. There are also those people who use a combination of ribs and diaphragm to varying degrees. A large proportion of folks are shallow breathers no matter which part of the respiratory apparatus they favor.

A full inhale will result in the expansion of the ribs and the diaphragm. The good exhale will relax both. Many people do not breathe into the upper ribs. This is especially true in NYC, where almost everyone has tight shoulders that restrict the upper ribs. Hence, the shoulders (and the arms) must relax and we often say: "Breathe into your shoulders." The exhale can allow the shoulders to relax so that the upper ribs can be felt and used with the next inhale.

A good exhale does not mean collapsing the chest—merely relaxing it. This has greater implications. To repeat, it's like jumping into cold water. At first the response is to gasp and hold the breath on the inhale. When an exhale finally can happen, the water doesn't seem so cold. There is the same tendency to hold the breath on the inhale in physical or emotional pain; the exhale can be used to relieve some of that pain.

The effect of the diaphragm in abdominal breathing is the expansion of the belly. Many people (especially Yoga breathers) accomplish this by pushing out the front of the abdomen. This can result in a shortening of the lower back with inhalation. Unfortunately, this may eventually cause poor posture and lower back pain.

A more functional view of abdominal breathing is to allow the breath response to extend down into the pelvic bowl. The pelvic diaphragm is the bottom of the abdomen (many people are very surprised to learn this). This allows for a lengthening of the area between the respiratory and pelvic diaphragms, causing the person to straighten and lengthen.

As Rolfers, we believe that breathing into an area allows more awareness there. By promoting such awareness in the pelvis, we often run into cultural inhibitions. Simply put, it is not O.K. to feel that part of your body, period. Yet secretly, people long to do so. People love it when I tell them that they can feel their pelvis and nobody else will know. Once the inhibition of feeling with the breath in that area is overcome, the smiles become more heartfelt and "sexfelt."

A Guide to Self Control ... Mormon Style

[This text is an example of religious and cultural conservatism]

OVERCOMING MASTURBATION
distributed by Latter Day Science Church at Brigham Young University

The attitude a person has toward his problem has an effect on how easily it is overcome. It is essential that a firm commitment be made to control the habit. As a person understands his reasons for the behavior, and is sensitive to the conditions or situations that may trigger a desire for the act, he develops the power to control it.

We are taught that our bodies are temples of God, and are to be clean so that the Holy Ghost may dwell within us. Masturbation is a sinful habit that robs one of the Spirit and creates guilt and emotional stress. It is not physically harmful unless practiced in the extreme. It is a habit that is totally self-centered, and secretive, and in no way expresses the proper use of the procreative power given to man to fulfill eternal purposes. It therefore separates a person from God, and defeats the gospel plan.

This self-gratifying activity will cause one to lose his self-respect and feel guilty and depressed, which can in the extreme lead to further sinning. As a person feels spiritually unclean, he loses interest in prayer, his testimony becomes weak, and missionary work and other Church callings become burdensome, offering no joy and limited success.

To help in planning an effective program to overcome the problem, a brief explanation is given of how the reproductive organs in a young man function.

The testes in your body are continuously producing hundreds of millions of reproductive cells called spermatozoa. These are moved up a tube called the vas deferens to a place called the ampulla, where they are mixed with fluids from two membranous pouches called seminal vesicles and the prostate gland. The resultant fluid is called semen. When the seminal vesicles are full a signal is sent to the central nervous system indicating they are ready to be emptied. The rate at which this filling takes place varies greatly from one person to another, depending on such things as diet, exercise, state of health, etc. For some it may be several times a week, for others twice a month, and for others hardly ever.

It is normal for the vesicles to be emptied occasionally at night during sleep. This is called a "wet dream." The impulses that cause the emptying come from the central nervous system. Often an erotic dream is experienced at the same time, and is part of the normal process. If a young man has constantly masturbated instead of letting nature take its course, the reproductive system is operating at a more rapid pace, trying to keep up with the loss of semen. When he stops the habit, the body will continue to produce at this increased rate for an indefinite period of time, creating sexual tensions and pressure. These are not harmful and are to be endured until the normal central nervous system's pathway of release is once again established.

During this period of control several things can be done to make the process easier and more effective. As one meets with his priesthood leader, a program for overcoming masturbation can be implemented using some of the suggestions which follow. Remember it is essential that a regular report program be agreed on, so progress can be recognized and failures understood and eliminated.

SUGGESTIONS

1. Pray daily, ask for the gifts of the Spirit, that which will strengthen you against temptation. Pray fervently and out loud when the temptations are the strongest.

2. Follow a program of vigorous daily exercise. These exercises reduce emotional tensions and depression and are absolutely basic to the solution of this problem. Double your physical activity when you feel stress increasing.

3. When the temptation to masturbate is strong, yell stop to those thoughts as loudly as you can in your mind and then recite a pre-chosen scripture or sing an inspirational hymn. It is important to turn your thoughts away from the selfish need to indulge.

4. Set goals of abstinence, begin with a day, then a week, month, year, and finally commit to never doing it again. Until you commit yourself to never again, you will always be open to temptation.

5. Change in behavior and attitude is most easily achieved through a changed self-image. Spend time every day imagining yourself strong and in control, easily overcoming tempting situations.

6. Begin to work daily on a self-improvement program. Relate this plan to improving your church service, to improving your relationships with your family, God and others. Strive to enhance your strengths and talents.

7. Be outgoing and friendly. Force yourself to be with others and learn to enjoy working and talking with them. Use principles of developing friendships found in books such as *How to Win Friends and Influence People* by Dale Carnegie.

8. Be aware of situations that depress you or that cause you to feel lonely, bored, frustrated, or discouraged. These emotional states can trigger the desire to masturbate as a way of escape. Plan in advance to counter these low periods through various activities, such as reading a book, visiting a friend, doing something athletic, etc.

9. Make a pocket calendar for a month on a small card. Carry it with you, but show it to no one. If you have a lapse of self-control color that day black. Your goal will be to have no black days. The calendar becomes a strong visual reminder of self-control and should be looked at when you are tempted to add another black day. Keep your calendar up until you have at least three clear months.

10. A careful study will indicate you have had the problem at certain times and under certain conditions. Try and recall, in detail, what your particular times and conditions were. Now that you understand how it happens, plan to break the pattern through counter-activities.

11. In the field of psychotherapy there is a very effective technique called aversion therapy. When we associate or think of something very

distasteful with something which has been pleasurable, but undesirable, the distasteful thought and feeling will begin to cancel out that which was pleasurable. If you associate something very distasteful with your loss of self-control it will help you stop the act. For example, if you are tempted to masturbate think of having to bathe in a tub of worms, and eat several of them as you do the act.

12. During your toilet and shower activities leave the bathroom door or shower curtain partly open, to discourage being alone in total privacy. Take cool brief showers.

13. Arise immediately in the mornings. Do not lie in bed awake, no matter what time of day it is. Get up and do something. Start each day with an enthusiastic activity.

14. Keep your bladder empty. Refrain from drinking large amounts of fluids before retiring.

15. Reduce the amount of spices and condiments in your food. Eat as lightly as possible at night.

16. Wear pajamas that are difficult to open, yet loose and not binding.

17. Avoid people, situations, pictures or reading materials that might create sexual excitement.

18. It is sometimes helpful to have a physical object to use in over-coming this problem. A Book of Mormon, firmly held in hand, even in bed at night has proven helpful in extreme cases.

19. In very severe cases it may be necessary to tie a hand to the bed frame with a tie in order that the habit of masturbating in a semi-sleep con-dition can be broken. This can also be accomplished by wearing several layers of clothing which would be difficult to remove while half-asleep.

20. Set up a reward system for your successes. It does not have to be a big reward. A quarter in a receptacle each time you overcome or reach a goal. Spend it on something which delights you and will be a continu-ing reminder of your progress.

21. Do not let yourself return to any past habit or attitude patterns which were part of your problem. Satan never gives up. Be calmly and confidently on guard. Keep a positive mental attitude. You can win this fight! The joy and strength you will feel when you do will give your whole life a radiant and spiritual glow of satisfaction and fulfillment.

STEPS IN OVERCOMING MASTURBATION

Be assured that you can be cured of your difficulty. Many have been, both male and female, and you can be also if you determine that it must be so.

This determination is the first step. That is where we begin. You must decide that you will end this practice, and when you make that decision, the problem will be greatly reduced at once.

But it must be more than a hope or a wish, more than knowing that it is good for you. It must be actually a DECISION. If you truly make up your mind that you will be cured, then you will have the strength to resist any tendencies which you may have and any temptations which may come to you.

After you have made this decision, then observe the following specific guidelines:

1. Never touch the intimate parts of your body except during normal toilet processes.

2. Avoid being alone as much as possible. Find good company and stay in this good company.

3. If you are associated with other persons having this same problem, YOU MUST BREAK OFF THEIR FRIENDSHIP. Never associate with other people having the same weakness. Don't suppose that two of you will quit together, you never will. You must get away from people of that kind. Just to be in their presence will keep your problem foremost in your mind. The problem must be taken OUT OF YOUR MIND for that is where it really exists. Your mind must be on other and more wholesome things.

4. When you bathe, do not admire yourself in a mirror. Never stay in the bath more than five or six minutes—just long enough to bathe and dry and dress AND THEN GET OUT OF THE BATHROOM into a room where you will have some member of your family present.

5. When in bed, if that is where you have your problem for the most part, dress yourself for the night so securely that you cannot easily touch your vital parts, and so that it would be difficult and time-consuming for you to remove those clothes. By the time you started to remove protective clothing, you would have sufficiently controlled your thinking that the temptation would leave you.

6. If the temptation seems overpowering while you are in bed, GET OUT OF BED AND GO INTO THE KITCHEN AND FIX YOURSELF A SNACK, even if it is in the middle of the night, and even if you are not hungry, and despite your fears of gaining weight. The purpose behind this suggestion is that you GET YOUR MIND ON SOMETHING ELSE. You change the subject of your thoughts, so to speak.

7. Never read pornographic material. Never read about your problem. Keep it out of your mind. Remember—"first a thought, then an act." The thought pattern must be changed. You must not allow this problem to remain in your mind. When you accomplish that, you soon will be free of the act.

8. Put wholesome thoughts into your mind at all times. Read good books—Church books, scriptures, sermons of the brethren. Make a daily habit of reading at least one chapter of scripture, preferably from one of the four gospels in the New Testament, or the *Book of Mormon.* The four gospels—Matthew, Mark, Luke and John—above anything else in the Bible can be helpful because of their uplifting qualities.

9. Pray. But when you pray, don't pray about this problem, for that will tend to keep it in your mind more than ever. Pray for faith, pray for understanding of the scriptures, pray for the missionaries, the General Authorities, your friends, your families, BUT KEEP THE PROBLEM OUT OF YOUR MIND BY NOT MENTIONING IT EVER—NOT IN CON-VERSATION WITH OTHERS, NOT IN YOUR PRAYERS. KEEP IT OUT of your mind!

reprints: The Utah Liberation Army, P.O. Box 11563, Salt Lake City, Utah 84147

References

Bordo, Susan. *The Male Body: A New Look at Men in Public and in Private.* New York: Farrar, Straus and Giroux, 1999.

Brash, James Cooper. *Cunningham's Textbook of Anatomy,* 9th ed. London: Oxford University Press, 1953.

Chia, Mantak, and Arava, D. A. *The Multi-Orgasmic Man.* New York: Harper Collins, 1996.

Crelin, Edmund S. *Anatomy of the Newborn: An Atlas.* Philadelphia: Lea & Febiger, 1969.

Danielou, Alain. *The Phallus: Sacred Symbol of Male Creative Power.* Rochester, VT: Inner Traditions International, 1995.

Gore, Margaret. *The Penis Book: An Owner's Manual.* St. Leonards, NSW, Australia: Allen & Unwin, 1997.

Gorman, David. *The Body Moveable,* vol. 1. London: David Gorman, 1981.

Griffin, Gary. *Penis Size and Enlargement: Facts, Fallacies, and Proven Methods.* Aptos, CA: Hourglass Book Publishing, 1995.

Kegel, Arnold H. "Stress Incontinence and Genital Relaxation," *CIBA Clinical Symposium,* vol. 1 (2): 35-52, 1952.

Latey, Philip. "Feelings, Muscles and Movement," *Journal of Bodywork and Movement Therapies* (1): 44-52, 1996.

Lockhart, R. D., Hamilton, G. F., and Fyfe, F. W. *Anatomy of the Human Body.* Philadelphia: J. B. Lippincott, 1959.

Morganstern, Steven, and Abrahams, Allen. *Overcoming Impotence.* Englewood Cliffs, NJ: Prentice Hall, 1994.

Morin, Jack. *Anal Pleasure and Health.* San Francisco: Yes Press, 1981.

Netter, Frank H. *Atlas of Human Anatomy.* Summit, NJ: Ciba-Geigy Corp., 1989.

Pernkoff, Eduard. *Atlas of Topographical and Applied Human Anatomy*, vol 2. Philadelphia & London: W. B. Saunders Co., 1964.

Schultz, R. Louis, and Feitis, Rosemary. *The Endless Web.* Berkeley: North Atlantic Books, 1996.

Schwartz, Kit. *The Male Member.* New York: St. Martin's Press, 1985.

Strage, Mark. *The Durable Fig Leaf.* New York: William Morrow & Co., Inc., 1980.

Van Howe, Robert S., ed. *Circumcision,* vol. 1, #1, June 1995.

Zilbergeld, Bernie. *Male Sexuality.* Boston-Toronto: Little, Brown and Company, 1978.

Index